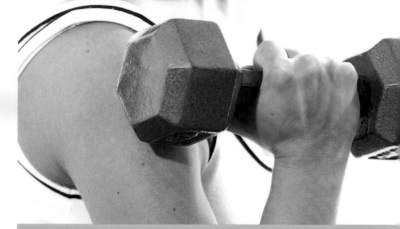

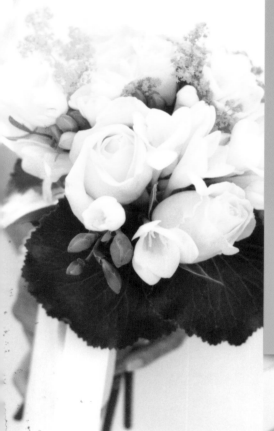

THE

healthy
BRIDE GUIDE

BE FIT *and* FABULOUS
FROM THIS
DAY FORWARD

Christi Masi
with SHERI MAR

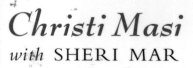

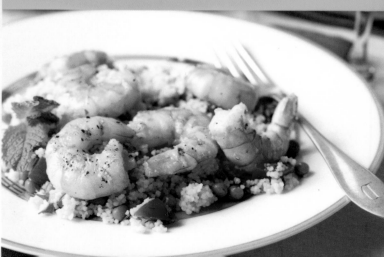

The healthy BRIDE GUIDE

Be fit and fabulous from this day forward

CHRISTI MASI

SASQUATCH
BOOKS

This book is dedicated to my husband Scott, my dear friends Marilyn and Lisa, and to all healthy brides on their wondrous wedding day.

Printed in Canada
Published by Sasquatch Books
Distributed by Publishers Group West
12 11 10 09 08 07 06 05   10 9 8 7 6 5 4 3 2 1

Interior design and composition: Stewart A. Williams
Interior illustrations: Leela Corman / www.glittercannon.com
Cover design: Nina Barnett
Cover photographs:
   Weights © Albert Normandin / Masterfile
   Bouquet © Hiep Vu / Masterfile
   Food © Melanie Acevedo / PictureArts / CORBIS
Author photograph: Annie Marie Musselman

Library of Congress Cataloging-in-Publication Data is available.

ISBN 1-57061-461-X

Sasquatch Books
119 South Main Street, Suite 400
Seattle, WA 98104
(206) 467-4300
www.sasquatchbooks.com
custserv@sasquatchbooks.com

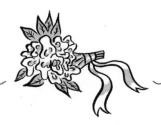

Contents

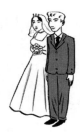

Acknowledgments

Many thanks to the following who generously spent time answering my many, many questions.

Jamie Hsu, *Ethereal Events*

Karen Guyt, *Studio G Occasions*

Sheri Miller, *Esprit de Fleur*

Evette from *Brides by Dimetrio*

Charity from *Marcellas La Boutique*

Vicky Grayland, *Grayland photography*

Lindsay Anderson, *Lindsay wedding photography*

Jennifer Heidal Wiley

Jennifer Bates

Catherine Martin

Vickie from *Ravishing Radish*

Judy Heidal

Valerie Corcoran, MSW

Introduction

Life is a terrific journey filled with joy, responsibility, challenge, and relationships. None of the fun would exist without the others you share your precious life moments with. My friends, family, and coworkers have always been very important to me, and as I get older I realize that the most valuable assets in my life are the relationships I have with these people. I also recognize that before I can have healthy relationships with them, I must start by having a healthy relationship with myself.

Many of you are planning for your wedding and readying yourself for your new life with your fiancé. This book is meant to serve as a how-to guide for developing the most important relationship in your life—the one you have with yourself. If you don't have a healthy relationship with yourself, the relationships you have with others will not be as enjoyable, responsible, challenging, or deep. Taking care of yourself is not optional; it's mandatory.

My goal in writing *The Healthy Bride Guide* has been to provide brides, their friends, and their families with a guide for healthful living through fitness, food, and stress management that is easy to follow and easy to incorporate into your life. I've tried to make this book—and the program it outlines—as enjoyable as possible. We all know that healthy living has to involve at least a little fun for you to stick with it.

The purpose of this book is to help women at a pivotal point in their lives to choose a healthy lifestyle from now on. Change is hard, especially when it comes to taking care of yourself. Women are particularly bad at putting themselves first. We seem to have inherited a gene that programs us to take care of everyone else first. I want to reprogram this gene so that it tells women, "Take care of yourself first, and then you'll be better able to take care of the other people in your life." Planning a wedding and embarking on a marriage offers you a special opportunity to look at your own health and decide that you are worth it, and that you deserve to be the best you possible.

The Healthy Bride program employs a simple format that will assist you in choosing a healthy lifestyle. I have structured the book to help you take small steps toward making changes that can last a lifetime. I believe in lifelong results, not short-term fixes. Remember, you are making a lifetime commitment to your marriage. And what better time to make the same level of commitment to yourself.

My aim is to help you make this commitment to your health as easy as possible. The first part of the book will help you assess how healthy you are and whether you are really, truly ready to change. I then lay out a fitness program that features an exercise progression you can move through slowly, advancing only as you are ready. Next, Sheri Mar, a licensed nutritionist and longtime colleague of mine, details a healthy eating program for you.

The book also features a stress management program, something I know from experience is a necessity during the anxiety-ridden days leading up to a wedding. In this part of the book, you'll find a smorgasbord of tips, tricks, and sage advice from which you can pick and choose what you want to include in your own Bridal Stress Survival Kit. Finally, I offer an "after the honeymoon" program, which teaches you to incorporate these eating, exercise, and stress management habits into your new married life.

Each chapter will offer easy-to-follow steps to walk you through the Healthy Bride program. The book will help you assess where you are today in terms of healthy diet, exercise, and stress management and help you determine what type of workout, eating, and stress management routine makes the most sense for you. Then you'll learn how you can stay on track for months and years to come.

Throughout the book, we set goals to help you stay focused and measure your progress at specific points in time. The overall goal is to continue living a healthy, vibrant life long after you say your vows. We see your wedding day as a pivotal point in your life—and your health—not as an end point. In getting married, you're embarking on a new chapter in life. We're here to help you seize this opportunity to develop and maintain an ongoing healthy lifestyle so that you can live the life you truly want to live . . . from this day forward.

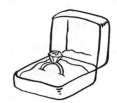

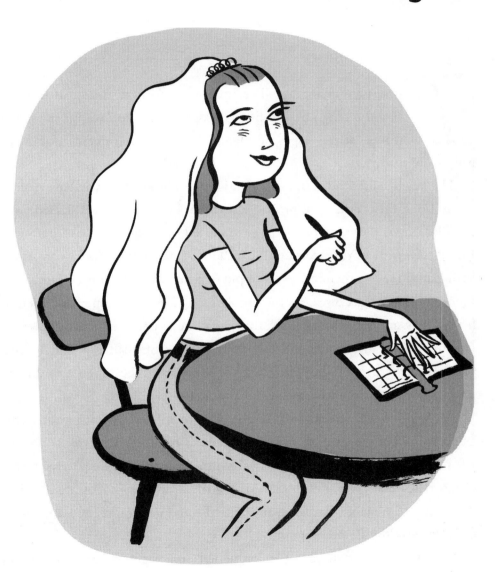

You are about to embark upon a new life.

Things are changing all around you, and now is a great time to begin a new physical fitness program. Are you ready? Let's take a look at the stages of change. Then you can decide if you are really, truly ready.

The key to a lifetime of fitness is consistency. The fact that you have picked up this book means that you probably have not been able to get started with a regular fitness program, or if you have started one, you may have not been able to stay with it. You are not alone. Only 25 percent of American adults participate in recommended levels of physical activity, which is certainly not a good statistic. Heart disease is the number-one killer of women and men in this country, and for many people, this tragic life experience is avoidable.

This part of the book will discuss the stages of change and help you determine where you fall in The Stages of Motivation Readiness for Change Model continuum, as discussed in Chapter 1.

We will ask you to take some tests and to look deep into yourself to determine whether you are ready to adopt a healthier lifestyle. Next, we will review your current state of health using our wellness and risk factor inventories. Finally, we will set SMART goals—aspirations that are Specific, Measurable, Attainable, Realistic, and Timed—and get you ready for exercise using the Healthy Bride program.

You will want to have a pen or pencil and paper ready while going through this chapter. Take your time, be honest, and be thoughtful. What you end up writing down may surprise you.

CHAPTER 1

Stages of Change and Physical Activity

According to The Stages of Motivational Readiness for Change Model, individuals move through a series of stages as they adopt and maintain a new habit (Prochaska and DeClemente 1983). This model was determined after researchers studied groups of people participating in smoking and alcohol cessation programs and monitored how they moved through the behavior change process. The model has been validated and applied to a variety of behaviors, including smoking cessation, exercise, contraceptive use, and diet.

Behavioral change is rarely a casual, single event. The Stages of Change model shows that, for most people, a change in behavior occurs gradually (you didn't decide to get married overnight, for example), with the person moving from being uninterested, unaware, or unwilling to make a change (known as the precontemplation stage) to considering a change (the contemplation stage) to deciding and preparing to make a change.

Making a change in life requires purposeful, determined action. This does not come without planning, dedication, effort, and a great desire. Relapses are a normal part of change and should not come as a surprise; they are just part of the change process. Many people find themselves moving cyclically through these stages before the change becomes established.

Let's look at the stages and determine where you fall. Specifically, these stages, as applied to exercise, include:

1. **Precontemplation.** You are not even considering exercise, let alone scheduling it in your weekly routine.

2. **Contemplation.** You regularly consider beginning to exercise, but you make no effort to incorporate exercise into your schedule.

3. **Preparation.** You are working out, but not at recommended levels. Your exercise times are also inconsistently scheduled or not scheduled at all.

4. **Action.** You are exercising at recommended levels, but have done so for less than six months.

5. **Maintenance.** You have been exercising regularly and on schedule at recommended levels for more than six months.

Most people move through these stages at different points in their lives. The movement tends to be cyclical rather than linear; you move through the stages in an orbital fashion.

You can also look at these stages in the context of maintaining healthy eating habits. Because the two topics go hand in hand, when you examine your fitness program, you also should assess your eating habits. Otherwise, you're not going to be as healthy as you could. Looking at both areas of your well-being will give you a truer picture of where you stand today. In fact, you may find you score better in one area than the other.

Before you move on, go back through the previous list, substituting "healthy eating" for "exercise" throughout to determine what stage of maintaining a nutritious, healthy diet you are in. This will also prepare you for the questionnaire on the following page.

Physical Activity Stages of Change Questionnaire

Take this brief test to see what stage you are in. For each of the following statements, please circle Y or N. Please be sure to read each statement carefully and to answer truthfully.

For all statements, being physically active includes activities such as walking briskly, jogging, bicycling, swimming, or any other activity in which exertion is at least as intense as these activities.

1. I consider myself currently physically active.   **Y/N**

2. I intend to become more physically active in the next six months.   **Y/N**

For the next two statements, for physical activity to be "regular," it must add up to a total of 30 minutes or more per day and be done at least five days per week. For example, you could take one 30-minute walk or three 10-minute walks for a daily total of 30 minutes.

3. I currently engage in regular physical activity.   **Y/N**

4. I have been regularly physically active for the past six months.   **Y/N**

Scoring

Now look at your responses to the four statements and identify which stage matches you. Read the section of text in the following pages that applies to your stage.

Precontemplation: Statement 1 = no; statement 2 = no

Contemplation: Statement 1 = no; statement 2 = yes

Preparation: Statement 1 = yes; statement 3 = yes; statement 4 = no

Action: Statement 1 = yes; statement 3 = yes; statement 4 = no

Maintenance: Statement 1 = yes; statement 3 = yes; statement 4 = yes

Which stage are you currently in? _____

Source: ADAPTED FROM MARCUS, BANSPACH, LEFEBVRE, ROSSI, CARLETON, AND ABRAMS 1992.

Precontemplation

If you are in this stage, you are probably not too interested in this book and may just be glossing over it. Maybe this book was a gift from a cruel but concerned family member or friend. But as long as I have your attention, let's put together a quick list of the pros and cons of exercise. Physical activity yields so many benefits that to not do it really is to ignore your health. Many people could improve their health, spirit, energy, and quality of life if only they would exercise.

Here are the pros and cons of exercise I generally hear from the brides I work with:

Pros	**Cons**
I feel healthier.	I don't have any time.
I have more energy.	I hate all forms of exercise.
Exercising helps me reduce stress.	I don't like to sweat.
Exercising helps me sleep better.	I'm too old.
I can move more easily and have more flexibility.	I'm too out of shape.
I am stronger.	I have no energy for exercise.

As you can see, the pros far outweigh the cons. With help, support, and encouragement, the precontemplative person can move to the contemplative stage. For those who "hate" exercise or feel they may be physically limited, there is a form of exercise for all levels of capability, whether it's rowing, walking, gardening, kickboxing, belly dancing, or ballroom dancing. Exercise does not have to be a daunting, painful experience maintained for a sweating, lung-burning 45 minutes to give you results; even moderate activity can make a tremendous difference. Every 10 minutes counts, and starting out slowly is smart.

Furthermore, I don't buy the "I don't have time" argument because people seem to have plenty of time in their lives for television. Take some of that TV time and turn it into something productive. It's about setting priorities and including activity in your daily life. Before you know it, your exercise and healthy eating program will be making a difference in your life.

Hopefully you're now motivated enough to enter the contemplation stage. Go on and read the next section. You'll feel better about yourself.

Contemplation

If you're at this stage, that may be why you picked up this book. Thank yourself for being here. You have probably made a list of exercise pros and cons and are wondering what to do next. You are the ideal reader for this book and the reader for whom I outlined the Level One stage in Chapter 8 of the fitness section (Part Two). After reading the remaining chapters in this part of the book, you should begin your exercise program by turning to the fitness section and reading my recommendations.

Start slowly and try not to take an all-or-nothing approach to your new exercise program. If you miss a day or two, don't worry. Just keep marching forward. Do what you can, experiment with various modes of exercise, and find which activities you like best. Small changes count. Make sure you reward yourself for the little victories such as taking the stairs instead of an elevator and walking further to work each day from your bus stop. Keep setting small, achievable goals, keep telling yourself that doing something is better than doing nothing, and hang in there.

Sometimes the best way to ensure you stick with it is to find a workout buddy. Social support and accountability make a huge difference in people's ability to stay on track with their exercise program.

Preparation

Congratulations to you if you fall into this stage. You are well on your way to a lifetime of fitness. Although you are still trying to get into your routine, you understand the benefits of exercise. Two words of advice: Don't stop! Keep exercising, and stay focused on your plan and on the activities you like to do. Your goal should be to do more of what you're currently doing.

The fitness section of this book (Part Two) contains workout plans and schedules that may help you. You are the best person to determine what level of exercise suits you. Start from where you are today, and don't push too hard. For example, if you are exercising three times per week but are not doing any resistance training, continue with your three days and add one day of resistance training. Review the exercise programs in this book, look for the schedule that most closely matches your current exercise program, and progress from there. Stay on the path you feel comfortable with, and don't do too much. The key to your success is to set small, measurable goals and to celebrate your successes when you achieve them.

Action and Maintenance

If you fall into either of these groups, you're in that 25 percent mentioned earlier. Good job! The key word for you now is *maintain*. You are doing very well and it's important you keep going. Use Part Two of this book, the exercise section, for help with your physical fitness program, and be sure you are setting and resetting your goals at approximately six-week intervals. You may find some of the lower-intensity exercise levels in Part Two too easy. Feel free to bump yourself up a level or two, as long as you maintain a comfort level with your program. Whatever you do, don't get too ambitious and push yourself beyond your limits.

In addition, think ahead to how you will maintain your workouts during vacations, illness, and boredom. You already are doing great and just need to practice some positive self-talk down the road in the event that you encounter any bumps. Congratulations for prioritizing exercise in your life. Now the trick is to focus on keeping it a priority in the long run. Before beginning to polish your exercise routine, read the next section on how to handle a possible backslide in your workout program.

Buck the Backslide Kit

Those of you in the later stages of making a change, particularly the action and maintenance stages, should put together a list of steps you will take if and when you're faced with a lapse in your desire to continue your exercise and healthy eating program—what we will call a "backslide." The reason for creating this kit now is so that you have it ready to pull out later when you need it. You can put it to use when your exercise program is not going as well as it is now. Having written the plan while maintaining your current level of commitment will give you a positive perspective (in your own voice) that can help pull you out of a backslide.

Your Buck the Backslide Kit should include these items:

• Three favorites from your Bridal Stress Survival Kit (see
  page 196)

- A list of your big goals (see page 15) for your life (not the short-term ones)

- A written statement about why you wanted to change in the first place and why exercise is important to you

- A few sentences that will resound with you, written in your "new voice"—that is, the voice that's excited and motivated to develop a new, healthier lifestyle

Put this kit where you can find it later when you need it most. When you begin to backslide, pull this kit out and remind yourself why you are making this change and what it means to you. This will remind you of how good you were feeling when your exercise program was going well. We discuss your Buck the Backslide Kit in more detail in Part Five (Beyond Bridal).

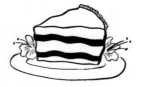

CHAPTER 2

Taking Your Health Inventory

Y ou can exercise your way to better health by paying attention to certain risk factors and determining which affect you. As this chapter describes, some of these risk factors will affect the type of exercise program you embark on. Some of these items are not at your will to change. However, some are, so you may want to see what you can do to curb these risks.

Risk Factors for Coronary Heart Disease

There are some risk factors you cannot change, such as your age, gender, and heredity.

- **Increasing age.** Most people who die of heart attack are more than 65 years old, but cardiovascular disease can strike at any time in life.

- **Gender.** Heart disease is the number one killer of women. Men have a higher risk as a gender, but the risk of heart attack for women increases after menopause, closing the gap to become equal to the risk for men.

- **Heredity.** Children of parents with heart disease are more likely to develop heart disease themselves.

However, there are other factors you can control. Ask yourself if any of the following apply to you:

- **Smoking.** Do you smoke?

- **Cholesterol.** Is your total serum cholesterol level greater than 200 mg/dl? Is your HDL (the good cholesterol) less than 40 mg/dl? (mg/dl = milligrams per deciliter)

- **High blood pressure.** Is your blood pressure higher than 140/90?

- **Diabetes mellitus.** Is your fasting blood sugar level 100–125 mg/dl or more?

- **Physical activity.** Do you exercise rarely or not at all?

- **Weight management.** Is your Body Mass Index (BMI) more than 30?

To figure out whether the final risk in this list (obesity) applies to you, you need to know your Body Mass Index. To do this, follow the instructions in the "BMI Calculation" sidebar on page 13.

What Are Your Risks?

Look at the list of risk factors in the previous section and figure out where you are on the risk factor scale.

- If you answered yes to one or more of these risk factor questions, then you are considered at increased risk for heart disease. The more risk factors you have, the higher your risk. Please see your doctor to get a thorough evaluation.

BMI Calculation

TO DETERMINE YOUR BMI, you need to first convert your height and weight to metric units. For the following explanation, let's use the example of a woman who is 5 feet 5 inches and weighs 115 pounds.

1. Take your height in inches and multiply that by .0254. The result is your height in meters. Using our example, we would first convert 5 feet 5 inches to inches, which gives us 65 inches. Then we multiply by .0254, giving us this equation: 65 inches x .0254 = 1.651 meters

2. Convert your weight in pounds to kilograms by dividing your weight by 2.2. Returning to our example:

   115 pounds / 2.2 = 52.27 kilograms

3. Take your weight in kilograms and divide it by the square of your height in meters. The end result is your BMI. Here is the equation using our example:

52.27 kilograms / (1.651 meters x 1.651 meters) = BMI of 19.1

Now that you know your BMI, which of these categories do you fall into?

Underweight: BMI of less than 18.5

Normal weight: 18.5–24.9 BMI

Overweight: 25–29.9 BMI

Obese: 30 or more

The BMI number is not perfectly accurate. Because it is based on large numbers of people and general population data, it cannot take into account specifics about your particular body. However, this number will give you an idea of where you are today, as compared to the general population.

• If you are not sure where you stand with regard to some of these risk factors, get a full checkup from your doctor to evaluate your risk level.

Source: AMERICAN HEART ASSOCIATION

No matter where you fall in this list, please see your doctor before beginning any exercise program. Bring this information to your physician's office and discuss what you can do to improve your health.

Reducing Risk Factors for Myocardial Infarction (Heart Attack)

You can make many changes in your lifestyle to help reduce your heart's health risk level:

- **Quit cigarette smoking**

  50–70% decrease in risk to your health within 5 years

- **Decrease blood cholesterol**

  2–3% decrease for each 1% drop in cholesterol (for people with elevated levels)

- **Decrease high blood pressure**

  2–3% decrease for each 1 mm Hg (mm Hg = millimeters of mercury) drop in diastolic pressure (the bottom number in your blood pressure reading)

- **Increase physical activity**

  45% decrease for those who maintain an active lifestyle

- **Maintain an ideal body weight**

  35–55% decrease for those who are not obese (more than 20% higher than their ideal body weight; see BMI Calculation sidebar on page 13)

Source: MANSON, TOSTESON, RIDKER, ET AL. 1992.

CHAPTER 3

Setting Realistic Goals

There are no secrets to success. It is the result of preparation, hard work, and learning from failure.

COLIN POWELL

Now that you know what your willingness to change is and you have a better picture of how healthy you are, it's time to set some goals. This is an activity we will return to again and again, and one that's key to the success of any exercise program. You may want to start with a huge goal for your entire lifetime. These are some examples of big life goals:

- I want to be able to hike and bike for the rest of my life, and I will do whatever it takes to make that a reality.

- I want to be able to play tennis with my fiancé, his family, and someday, our children and grandchildren.

- I want to continue dancing until I am well into my eighties and nineties. I love dancing.

- Each year of my life, I want to be able to participate in one competitive athletic event that I set as a goal for myself.

Then break this bigger goal into smaller, manageable goals that you can tackle individually, set deadlines for, and celebrate when you succeed.

Setting SMART Goals

When setting the smaller goals, make sure they are SMART: Specific, Measurable, Attainable, Realistic, and Timed.

Specific. State exactly what you want to achieve, how you're going to do it, and when you want to accomplish it. To begin, set goals you can achieve within a week to a month. It's easy to give up on goals that take too long to reach. If you have a big goal, break it down into a series of smaller weekly or daily goals. After you achieve one of the smaller goals, move on to the next.

Measurable. A goal doesn't do you any good if you have no way of determining whether you've achieved it. "I want to feel better" isn't a very good goal because it's not specific and it's difficult to measure. "I want to work out 30 minutes each day" is a better goal because it's both specific and measurable.

Attainable. Ask yourself whether your goal is within reasonable reach. For instance, completing a marathon may not be an achievable goal if you've never run before. However, completing a shorter run such as a 5K may be attainable.

Realistic. This is your call. What is realistic to you may not be to someone else. Your objective has to be within the realm of your own believability. If you can't envision yourself doing it, you won't follow through.

Timed. A goal must have a target date, and this time frame must be realistic. If you want to be able to do 15 push-ups without resting but don't set a timeline for it, it won't be motivating. A deadline too far in the future is too easily put off. A goal that's set too close to the present is not only unrealistic, it's discouraging.

Goal Worksheet

The goal worksheet on page 17 gives instructions on what to provide for each section. Create your own goal worksheet (see page 18) with this sample.

LIFE GOAL:
This big goal sums up your overall health aspirations for your entire life—for example, "My goal is to still be hiking and biking when I am in my seventies."

INTERMEDIATE GOAL:
This is your current short-term goal—for example, "I want to decrease my body fat by x% in 24 weeks."

TASKS:	TIMING:	SELF-ASSESSMENT:
Research the best workout and eating program.	Week 1	Find a program that fits my timeline and schedule, is realistic, and fits my lifestyle and goal.
Begin the program.	Week 1–4	Make sure the program fits my lifestyle and is working, and make adjustments to ensure I succeed.
Work through the program; monitor the program at regular intervals.	Week 2–12	Every six weeks, do new body measurements and push-up tests so that I know I am on track.
Have final dress fitting.	Week 18	I made it! My measurements were right on target for this date.
Finish line!	Week 24	Maintain my program until my wedding day. Do final push-up test.

RESULTS:
- Found program I like and put the schedule in my book (Week 1).
- Found a program that is fun for me and gives me long-term results that will get me to my finish line.
- Met regularly with my food and fitness coach or buddies to stay on track. We talked about our workouts, our food programs, and how they were working for us.
- Did my six-week body composition measurements; found that I was right on track. Lost .5 in. at all three sites. Did 12 push-ups. And lost 1% body fat.
- Continued on my program and felt great.
- Continued checking my body comp measurements every six weeks to make sure I stay on track.
- At 24 weeks, I crossed the finish line! I succeeded, and I feel great.

LIFE GOAL:		

INTERMEDIATE GOAL:		

TASKS:	TIMING:	SELF-ASSESSMENT:

RESULTS:		

CHAPTER 4

Final Words Before You Begin

The key to a lifetime of fitness is consistency. Here are some tips to help you on your path to making exercise a habit:

• Choose an activity you enjoy.

• Tailor your program to your own fitness level. (See Part Two of the book for details.)

• Set realistic goals.

• Choose an exercise program that fits your lifestyle.

• Give your body a chance to adjust to your new routine.

• Don't get discouraged if you don't see immediate results. It takes time for your body to adjust and make changes. It took some time to get out of shape, and it will take some time to get (back) into shape. You should start seeing results in six weeks, but that will vary from person to person. Be kind to yourself, and hang in there.

• Don't give up if you miss a day; just get back on track the next day.

- Find a partner for a little motivation and fitness bonding.

- Build some rest days into your exercise schedule.

- Listen to your body. If you have difficulty breathing or experience faintness or prolonged weakness during or after exercise, consult your physician.

Before we move on to the fitness part of the book, I have a few recommendations. First, find a comfortable place to exercise, whether it's in your home, in your backyard, or at a gym. In addition, if you don't already have the following items, I recommended you purchase them:

- **Exercise ball.** Get a physio ball (these are the big, round, inflated balls you see in gyms and physical therapy offices) that fits you well. To determine a good fit, use the following scale:

YOUR HEIGHT	SIZE OF BALL
Up to 4 ft 10 in. tall	42 cm ball (16 in.)
From 4 ft 11 in. to 5 ft 7 in. tall	53–55 cm ball (21 in.)
From 5 ft 8 in. to 5 ft 11 in. tall	65 cm ball (25 in.)
At least 6 ft tall	75 cm ball (29 in.)

These measurements are approximate; they will vary depending on your leg length, body weight, and how full you inflate the ball. In general, while seated on the ball, your legs should be even with (or slightly above) your hips.

- **Dumbbells.** Begin with 3 lb, 5 lb, and 8 lb weights. You may want heavier weights as you progress through the exercises in this book. If you already are in the active or maintenance stages, you may find these weights too light. Progress as you feel ready.

- **Resistance bands.** Most of the exercises in Levels One and Two of the Healthy Bride fitness program recommend using bands. They are light, versatile, and portable.

- **Exercise mat.** Using a mat makes doing floor exercises (especially crunches and sit-ups) more comfortable.

- **Loose-fitting clothing.** This gives all your joints a maximum range of motion.

- **Good shoes.** Good-fitting, quality exercise shoes are key to remaining injury-free. You should replace your shoes every 6 to 12 months, depending on how much stress you put on them. Check with a good athletic shoe store in your city or town.

You can find these items in most fitness or sports equipment stores. Or you can purchase a full kit directly from my company. Just visit The Healthy Bride website at www.healthy-bride.com.

Part Two

The Healthy Bride
Fitness Program

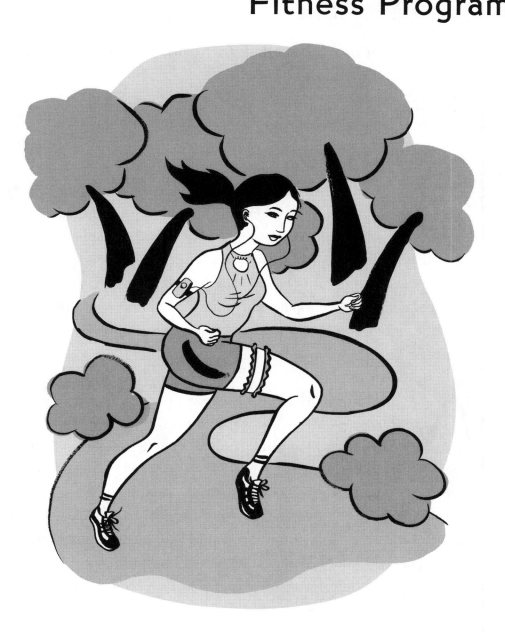

*Now that you're about to begin the
fitness portion of this program, you really need to
start showing that this will be a true commitment,
just as you will be committing yourself to marriage.*

As on your wedding day, you must vow to keep to this commitment:

Vows:

*I, _____ [state your name], take you, my body, to be my faith-
ful, healthy vessel of my life. I promise, from this day forward, that
I will honor you and cherish you. I will be faithful in your nourishment, exercise, and flexibility. And I will allow you to reach
your full potential, with full acceptance of your flaws, weaknesses,
and limitations. In sickness and in health, I promise to comfort
you, nurture you, and honor you for as long as we both shall live.*

Now that you have vowed to make this commitment, let's move
forward with *how* you will do this.

Exercise. You would think it was a four-letter word. We all
know we need to do it, yet many of us are loathe to. The U.S. Department of
Health and Human Services recommends being "physically active for at least
30 to 90 minutes on most days of the week"—brides-to-be included. Such
an amount of exercise will have you fit enough to sustain good health and
live a long life with your new husband. It's no longer just about you; it's also
about him. You not only owe it to yourself to maintain your health, you also

owe it to your life partner so that throughout your lives together you will be vibrant, active, healthy, and better able to face the challenges of everyday living. You will also have great health habits to pass along to your children, should you decide to start a family. With a commitment to health, all of you can lead healthier, more functional, and ultimately happier lives.

This part of the book focuses on which exercises and routines to do, when you should do them, how to do them, and how to get the most from each minute you work out. You will also learn how to integrate exercise into your life for the long term so that these habits last well beyond your wedding day. If a very busy bride like you can get motivated now, you can keep the momentum going . . . till death do you part.

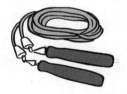

CHAPTER 5

The Elements of Exercise

To be healthy and lead a vibrant life you will want to have cardiovascular and muscular fitness, and you will want to be flexible. If you are strong enough to do the things you want, have the cardiovascular capacity to participate in the fun activities life offers, and have free-flowing joints that allow a full range of movement, your life will be fuller, richer, and more complete.

For example, say you are on your honeymoon and are staying on an exotic island. Your honey wants to go for a hike. You want to be fully prepared to go on that hike with him. First, you'll need to have the cardiovascular capacity to walk the trail and still enjoy the scenery along the way. Now suppose this hike leads to a beautiful pool with a waterfall dropping into it. You suspect the rocks by the waterfall would be an amazing place to canoodle with your honey. To get to that spot, you first would need to swing from a vine and drop into the pool. Then you'd need to swim over to the rocks near the waterfall. To do this, you'll need enough strength to hold on to that vine until it swings out over the middle of the pool. You'll also need the endurance to swim to those rocks near the waterfall. And to get onto those rocks, you'll need the flexibility to swing a leg up. With proper cardiovascular, strength, and flexibility training you can take that hike, swing that vine, swim to those rocks, and climb up them. And when you do, you will be rewarded by experiencing the warm, lovely waterfall up close with your husband.

This example may be a bit unlikely. But my point is that you never know what potential experiences life will offer, and to experience them fully you will need to have the proper cardiovascular, strength, and flexibility training. Consider these more common examples:

- Catching the bus at the bus stop before it pulls away. With good *cardiovascular* training, you will be able to make that 25-yard dash easily.

- Trying to get your garden prepared and planted before summer, including adding some dirt first. The *strength* you develop in this program will prepare you to move that dirt in record time.

- Being *flexible* enough to reach around to the back seat of your car to get the laptop you need for the meeting you are rushing to, without throwing out your back or shoulder.

All this exercise stuff is about living life more fully—and having a life that is continuously active, fun, and vibrant.

Let's Get FITT

Let's discuss some tools you will use to develop your exercise program. We'll begin with the FITT (Frequency, Intensity, Time, and Type) Principle. Using FITT's basic principles of exercise, I'll define the most important variables of exercise and combine them to create effective, results-driven programs for you. Here's a breakdown of each of these variables:

Frequency. How often you work out is significant. As mentioned, the U.S. Department of Health and Human Services recommends we include 30–90 minutes of physical activity (not just your workout time, but all activity; walking to work, vacuuming, yard work, and exercise contribute to this total each day) most days of the week. We all know how hard this is, so my recommendation is you commit to working out four days per week. If you work out more than four days a week, that's great—you get bonus points. Four days a week is hard enough for most folks, though. If you tell yourself, "I am going to work out every day between now and my wedding," and then fall short of this goal, you will feel bad. You may even quit working out altogether rather than face the dejection caused by failing to meet such a lofty goal. I want you to feel good and successful, which is why I recommend just four days.

Intensity. How hard you work your body also impacts the results you will achieve. The next chapter will discuss this area in further detail. I like to recommend two methods for gauging workout intensity. The first method is to use a heart-rate monitor. On page 36, I will step you through how to define your maximum heart rate (MHR) using a system more reliable than the chart hanging on the wall of your gym. The old 220-age formula (discussed on page 35) is too general to be very helpful. The second way to gauge your exercise intensity is to use the Rating of Perceived Exertion (RPE) scale. Your RPE measurement rates how hard you are working on a scale of 0-10. This is my preferred method for gauging workout intensity because it is easy and does not require any special equipment.

Time. How long you exercise makes a difference. Are you spending 5 minutes or 50 minutes? It's not only how long you are exercising that counts; you also want to consider how hard you work for that amount of time and how often you are doing the exercise. When you combine these three factors, you can then determine the effectiveness of your exercise program.

Type. The type of exercise you are doing matters, too. Are you swimming, biking, working on an elliptical trainer, doing resistance training, or all of the above? Variety is helpful in keeping your brain and body interested in exercise, and enjoying what you are doing is most important of all.

Three Categories of Fitness

As mentioned at the start of this chapter, the Healthy Bride program incorporates three categories of fitness: cardiovascular (or cardio), strength, and flexibility training.

Cardiovascular. This refers to all body functions relating to your heart, lungs, and circulatory system. Listen up, ladies: The number-one killer of women in our society is heart disease. That's right, heart disease—not breast cancer. Why do so many women die of this disease? For many reasons, but according to the American Heart Association, it's primarily because of high exposure to the major risk factors (listed on page 11 in Part One of the book) and the fact that women tend to ignore the risk factors they are most able to change. In the Starting Out section, you took a personal inventory of your health risk factors, so you should be aware of what you need to change. The best news about recognizing your risk factors is that you can do something about them. And the time to start reducing them is now.

Muscular strength and muscular endurance. *Muscular strength* is the amount of weight you can lift in one shot, while *muscular endurance* is how much weight you can lift over time. This program does not focus on either of these physical attributes specifically; instead, it uses resistance training to help you keep up with life's daily demands and to help keep your bones healthy and osteoporosis at bay. Bones build density only until you are about 30–35 years old; after that, they start to break down. A sedentary lifestyle can lead directly to bone loss, which is very hard to reverse. Being strong also makes life easier and more fun. Resistance training does not mean you will end up looking like a Neanderthal woman. Most women do not have enough testosterone to sprout the big muscles that men have, so don't worry about that. It is truly a great feeling to be strong enough to do the things you want to each day without fatigue, injury, or failure. When you are strong enough to do the things you want, you feel empowered and in control of your life.

Flexibility. Being flexible means you have the ability to move a joint through its complete range of motion. Maintaining range of motion allows you to carry out daily life activities with ease and enjoyment. Flexibility is very specific to the individual, and many variables contribute to it, including joint construction; muscle, tendon, ligament attachment locations; and past injuries. Being able to get your leg over your bike seat so that you can go for a ride and being able to reach into the back seat of the car without pain or injury is the type of flexibility this program focuses on. Stretching is best done after a workout. If you like to stretch prior to working out, be sure your muscles are warmed up first to help avoid injury. The easiest way to warm up is to walk briskly, jog, or bike for 5–10 minutes.

Additional Terminology

Here are a few more terms you will need to know for this exercise program:

Adaptation. Exercise puts stress on your body system. This stress is a good thing—it allows your muscles, cardiovascular system, and circulatory system to adapt to the change in physical activity. That is why you get stronger and more fit when you exercise. Your body is adapting. If, however, you were to do the same exercise routine every single day and did not add variety to your workouts, your body would no longer be stressed, and it would no longer adapt. When this happens, you're in maintenance mode. This is OK once you have reached the level of fitness you want to maintain, but if you are looking for change, you need to be sure you stress your body so it adapts.

Core. This refers to the trunk or torso region of your body. The Healthy Bride program focuses on strengthening the core first because it is the basis for every exercise you will do.

Interval training. This involves a repeated series of workouts, interspersed with rest periods. Interval training normally involves higher intensities of exercise to overload the cardiorespiratory system. You should not perform this type of training more than two times per week, and you should not do this type of training until you have been working out for a minimum of three months.

Pilates. The Pilates method is an exercise system focused on improving flexibility and strength for the entire body without building bulk. Pilates involves a series of controlled movements that engage your body and mind. I do not include specific Pilates methods in the Healthy Bride program, but Pilates is a great addition to any exercise program, especially for those brides looking to improve their core strength.

Reps. This signifies the number of times you move a weight or band up and down. The word "reps" is short for "repetitions."

Sets. This denotes the number of times you perform a series of reps of an exercise.

Spot reduction. This supposed theory suggests that to reduce specific areas of fat, you should concentrate on exercising only those areas. Contrary to what you have heard on TV and in magazines, this theory is false. *There is no such thing as losing fat through spot reduction.* Fat is lost throughout the body in a pattern dependent upon genetics, gender (actually, hormones), and age. You must reduce overall body fat to lose fat in any particular area. Although you lose or gain fat throughout the body, the last area to become lean and the first area to get fat seems to be the midsection (in men and some women) and the hips and thighs (in women and a few men). Sit-ups, crunches, leg-hip raises, leg raises, hip adduction, hip abduction, and the like will exercise only the muscles under the fat.

Yoga. There are two meanings associated with yoga. The first connotes a Hindu discipline aimed at training the consciousness to attain a state of perfect spiritual insight and tranquility. The second meaning is a system of exercises practiced as part of this Hindu discipline to promote control of the body and mind. I do not include specific yoga poses in the Healthy Bride program, but I love the practice as it improves flexibility and reduces stress.

CHAPTER 6

Fitness Tests for Setting Your Baseline

Getting started on your workout program and making sure it is as effective as possible will require you to do some testing. Have you ever watched people exercising away on a treadmill, an elliptical trainer, or a bike with not a hair out of place or even a trace of sweat on their brow? Well, those folks are not getting much from their workouts. Granted, what they are doing is better than sitting on the couch watching TV, but if they are working toward a goal or toward better health, they need to step things up a bit.

I'm not saying that the "no pain, no gain" philosophy is the only way to make a change. But you do need to stress your system so that it knows it needs to change. Why is this important? Because you want to get the most from each and every workout you do. You also want to be sure that what you are doing is helping you meet the goals you have set. You also need to know how much exercise is enough and how much is too much for you.

To know where you are headed fitness-wise, you need to know where you stand today. Have you ever tried to make an airline reservation without knowing the city you are departing from? Not likely. You need to know where you are starting from to get on a plane that will take you to your final destination. With an exercise plan, the principle is the same. To determine your starting point for this fitness program, you need to get a good picture of your current state of fitness and flexibility. The tests outlined in this chapter are measurements of where you are today in terms of cardiovascular and muscular strength, as well as endurance fitness. These tests will provide you with a baseline to compare your ongoing progress, and ultimately will help you determine the effectiveness of the program. We will not be comparing your scores to those of others. Our focus is on your improvement only.

To determine where to begin your cardio program, first review the Level One schedule. If you are already performing more cardio workouts per week than we have scheduled, read through the schedule until you identify the stage that most closely matches yours, and begin the program there. You may be at a different level with your cardio workouts than you are with your resistance training, and that is OK. Mix and match the levels to your current needs.

If you are beginning or are just getting back into the cardio program, please start with Level One and progress as you feel ready.

Cardiovascular Fitness Assessment: The Three-Minute Step Test

Determining cardiovascular fitness can be done in a number of ways, but to keep things simple, I've included the following heart-rate recovery test, the Three-Minute Step Test. This test was developed in the 1980s by the YMCA and is widely used to determine aerobic fitness. Today this test is considered among the best measurements of cardiovascular fitness available. It measures how quickly your heart rate returns to its resting level after a round of cardiovascular exercise. The closer your heart rate is to your resting rate after the three minutes of stepping, the better your cardiovascular fitness.

To begin: You will need a 12-inch step, a metronome, and a stopwatch. It is helpful (but not mandatory) to have a stethoscope for assistance in measuring your heart rate. If you do not have a stethoscope, make sure you practice finding your carotid or radial pulse prior to the test (see Finding Your Pulse sidebar on page 34).

You should be rested (no prior workout is permitted on this day), hydrated, and in workout clothing at the start of the test. The room should be at no more than 72°F and well ventilated. It also should have good lighting.

Finding Your Pulse

FOLLOW THESE instructions to find your pulse:

Radial pulse. Locate your pulse by placing your right index finger on the thumb side of your left wrist. Press lightly. You should feel a pulsing flow of blood. This pulsing is called the *radial pulse.* The radial artery is above the radius (the forearm bone on the thumb side). If you have difficulty locating your pulse on your wrist, then try the carotid pulse.

Carotid Pulse. Locate the *carotid pulse* by placing the index and middle fingers of your right hand on the side of your throat. Press your fingers to your Adam's apple until you feel your pulse.

The test: Set the metronome to 96 beats per minute. If you do not have a metronome, you can find one on the Internet at www.metronomeonline. com. Then follow the instructions on the site to play the virtual metronome over your speakers while conducting the test (or burn this pace onto a CD).

Set your stopwatch to three minutes. Step up onto the 12-inch step and then back down for the full three minutes, keeping to the beat of the metronome with each step. Right foot up, left foot up, right foot down, left foot down. Repeat. It is important to step with the beat at all times.

When three minutes are up, sit on the bench. Set the stopwatch for one minute and begin taking your pulse. Count your pulse at your radial or carotid site, or with a stethoscope. The pulse count should start immediately (within five seconds of ending your stepping) and continue for the full minute.

The results: Record your overall pulse count from the Three-Minute Step Test on the scorecard on page 42. We will do this test again and again to measure your cardiovascular fitness. What we want to see from your retests is for your pulse count to drop.

Monitoring Intensity: Maximum Heart Rate Tests and Rating of Perceived Exertion

You will use maximum heart rate (MHR) and Rating of Perceived Exertion (RPE) information to monitor intensity when working on your cardiovascular fitness throughout this program. As discussed in the previous chapter, your MHR is your heart rate at the highest intensity level your heart can reach, and your RPE measures how hard you are working on a scale of 0–10. The next few pages provide a number of tests that explain how to determine and use each of these measurements.

Maximum Heart Rate Tests

Heart rate is one way of noting your intensity level during exercise. Two methods to determine your MHR are provided here: a math test and a field test. Although determining MHR is a good measure, it requires a heart-rate monitor. Heart-rate monitors are available at most sporting goods stores. They can also easily be found online.

Math Test

This is a new test that you probably won't find in any gym yet. For years, many health professionals relied on the 220-age test to determine MHR. In that test, your MHR is determined by subtracting your age in years from the number 220. However, after lengthy testing funded by the National Institutes of Health, researchers at the University of Colorado confirmed suspicions that the 220-age formula overestimates rates for young adults and underestimates rates for older adults. So, they have proposed a new formula, 208 *minus* (0.7 *times* your age in years), which corrects the problems of the original formula.

For example, for a 35-year-old bride, the formula would read as follows:

208 - (.7 x 35) = 184 estimated maximum heart rate

The drawback to this method is that it gives only an estimate based on statistical averages and may not reflect your true heart rates. As with any mathematical system, there will be a margin of error. Because there is a bit of error in this system, I prefer to use the RPE scale (discussed on page 37).

Field Test to Determine Maximum Heart Rate

For a more personalized method of determining your heart rate, you may want to try the following test. *Only do this test if you have been working out for three months or more at a minimum of three days per week and have been cleared for unrestricted exercise by your doctor.*

Go out on the track wearing a heart-rate monitor and after a substantial warm-up, run as hard as you can. Watch the monitor for the highest number your heart rate goes to, or set your heart-rate monitor to record and store the highest number. The highest number probably reflects your maximum heart rate.

How to Use Maximum Heart Rate Information

Once you know your maximum heart rate, you can use percentages of this number to monitor your exercise intensity level. For example, if our hypothetical bride from the earlier math test wanted to work at a 40–60% intensity level, she would need to aim for a heart rate between 74 (184 x 40%) and 110 (184 x 60%) to maintain that intensity level.

Some machines have sensors that can monitor your heart-rate intensity level for you. The exercise schedules include RPE levels so that you know you are exercising at the right intensity to meet your goals.

In general, heart-rate levels are described by the following percentages of MHR:

Heart healthy: 40–60
Weight management: 60–70
Aerobic: 70–80
Anaerobic threshold: 80–90
Maximum: 90–100

Heart healthy. You are working at a level that improves your heart and will help your overall health and well-being for now. You will adapt to this level of exercise pretty quickly, and you are not burning many calories per hour.

Weight management. At this level, you are working hard enough to burn significant numbers of calories per hour; much of the fuel being used for your exercise is coming from fat. Total calorie burn counts most, so don't be tricked into staying at this level because you are burning a higher percentage of energy from fat.

Aerobic. Here you are working at an intensity level that will significantly improve your aerobic capacity, and you are at a high calorie-per-hour burn rate.

Anaerobic threshold. At this level, you are nearing your limit. You want to cross into this zone when doing interval training (starting in Level Two; discussed in Chapter 9), but you will not be able to stay here long.

Maximum. At this level, you are reaching your maximum heart rate. There is little reason to spend much time here, although you may touch this level with interval training.

Rating of Perceived Exertion

Another way to measure intensity is to use the Rating of Perceived Exertion (RPE) scale. Many experts believe that the RPE scale is a far better training tool, and it does not require expensive electronic gear. You probably know exactly how you feel when you put in maximum effort, such as when you sprint to the finish line of a foot race. The Rating of Perceived Exertion relates to heart rate and blood-oxygen exchange rate in a linear fashion. In other words, a higher Rating of Perceived Exertion indicates a higher heart rate and oxygen uptake—so no monitor is necessary.

Dr. Gunnar Borg introduced the field of perceived exertion in the 1950s. His RPE scale is used worldwide by professionals in medicine, exercise

Exercise Intensity Benefit Scale

Ratings	Description	Benefit
0	Lying on the couch watching TV	None
1	Am I exercising?	Better than nothing
2	Easy; no sweat	Helping your heart; you have to start somewhere
3	Between easy and hard; thinking of sweating	Some benefit; low calorie-per-minute burn rate
4	Moderate; some sweat	More benefit; moderate calorie-per-minute burn rate
5	Above moderate; nearing hard	Good place for long/endurance training
6	Hard; more sweat	Good workout if you sustain longer duration
7	Harder; feeling like work	Good workout; good level for improvement
8	Even harder; can't sustain this too long	Good workout; more stress so more improvement and calorie burn, but be careful
9	Getting close to maxing out; can hold this just a short time	Hard work; will not be able to maintain; OK to touch this level for variety, for improvement, and to burn megacalories, but be careful at this level
10	At my absolute maximum; no way I can hold this for any period of time	Don't go/stay here unless you are training at athlete level

physiology, psychology, cardiology, ergonomy, and sports. Many modifications have been made to the Borg Scale over the years; we will be using one of those modifications in the Healthy Bride program.

To determine your RPE rating any time you are exercising, use a scale of 0–10 and assign a number that matches how hard you are working. Next, look at the benefit scale on page 38 to see what benefits you are getting from your exercise.

Maximum Heart Rate vs. Rating of Perceived Exertion

Once you've monitored both your MHR and your RPE, choose the system that works best for you. I have used both methods of monitoring throughout the program, and I have cross-referenced the two systems for ease of use. Be aware that this is not a scientific reference guide but rather an anecdotal one that has been helpful to the brides I have worked with. (Call it Christi's Rating of Perceived Exertion Scale.)

Muscular Strength and Endurance Tests

In this program, we will focus on strength training for real-life movements. Most brides I work with want to look good, feel strong, and see their muscles develop or "tone up." I have yet to meet a bride who wants to look like a bodybuilder. This fitness program is designed to tone, strengthen, and develop full body fitness for life's activities.

To measure your progress as you work through the resistance-training program, you need to know your muscular strength and endurance capability today. Following are three simple strength tests to take at the start of the program to determine your starting point. You will repeat these tests at least three more times during the course of the program. What we want to see are increasing numbers as time goes on.

Perform the Three-Minute Step Test and all three fitness tests before beginning any of the exercise programs in this book, recording your results on the scorecard at the end of this chapter. You will use these tests to document your improvement. These tests are only for you to determine your progress. There is no reason to compare your results to those of anyone else. If you can do only one push-up, that's fine. The next time you perform these tests, I know you will do more—and that is the goal. Unless you have a fair amount of resistance-training experience, I recommend you begin at Level

Christi's Rating of Perceived Exertion Scale

RPE	Description	Percentage of MHR/effort
0	Nothing at all	0
.5	Very, very weak	20
1	Very weak	30
2	Weak	40
3	Moderate	50
4	Somewhat strong	60
5	Strong	70
6		75
7	Very strong	80
8		85
9		90
10	Very, very strong	100

One in the book's fitness program (discussed in Chapter 8) and progress from there. You want to be sure you are not overdoing it; start slowly and then progress.

Push-up Test

This test counts how many push-ups you can do at once.

To begin: For this test, having a second person present to count for you is beneficial. Get into the bent-knee push-up position—your back flat, knees on the floor, hands under shoulders. Make sure your back is rigid and in a straight line from your head to your knees.

The test: Your partner places his or her fist directly under your chest. Lower yourself down until you touch your partner's fist. Each time you touch your partner's fist, count that as one push-up. If you do not have a partner or don't want anyone else around, find an object the size of your fist (such as a potato, a small box, or a can) and use that instead. Just remember what object you use so that you can use the same one each time you retest yourself.

Do as many push-ups as you can, each time coming down to touch your counter's fist or the object you placed directly under your chest. Go until you cannot go any longer.

The results: Record this number on the scorecard at the end of this chapter for future comparison.

Sit-up Test

This test counts how many sit-ups you can do in one minute.

To begin: Lie on the floor with your knees bent and feet flat. Rest your hands on your thighs and secure your feet by a partner or under a chair or couch.

The test: Squeeze your abdominal muscles, push your back flat, and raise your torso high enough for your hands to touch the tops of your knees.

Fitness Test Scorecard

Use this scorecard to track your results in the tests given in this chapter.

SCORECARD	Base-line	Week 6	Week 12	Week 18	Week 24	Week 36	Week 42
Three-Minute Step Test							
Push-up Test							
Sit-up Test							
Squat Test							

Don't reach forward with your neck or head; just use your abdomen. Keep your lower back on the floor.

The results: Record this number on the scorecard above for future comparison.

Squat Test

This test measures how many squats you can do at once.

To begin: Stand in front of a chair with your feet approximately shoulder width apart, facing away from the chair as though you are about to sit down. The proper-sized chair to use is one that makes your knees form right angles when you are sitting.

The test: Squat down and lightly touch the chair with your derriere before standing back up. Do not sit all the way down. Do as many squats as you can without resting until you are fatigued.

The results: Write down the number of squats you did on the scorecard at the end of this chapter for future comparison.

Retesting

You will want to perform these tests every 6–8 weeks. Perform the tests using the same methodology each time. At each stage, check your progress before moving to the next level. Seeing and measuring your progress will be very motivating and will show you how much your hard work is paying off.

CHAPTER 7

Beginning the Healthy Bride Fitness Program

Now the fun begins! You have decided you are ready for this commitment and you have set your specific goals, so let's get started.

We are going to start slow to really, really set you up for success. The plan for the Level One phase of the workout program is to help you ease into this new commitment. Going slow may be hard to accept once you have made the decision to get into (or back into) shape. However, experience has shown me that the people who do the best are the ones who start slowly and build slowly. If you have been working out three times per week for more than three months, you may be able to skip Level One and go to the Level Two workout phase. My caution, however, before you jump ahead is to go slowly and give your body the time it needs to change. Remember, there are no quick-fix fitness programs that work and last.

Implementing Your Goals

Keep the goals you have set in mind as you work through this health program. Make sure that you break your goals down into smaller bites. I recommend that you start out with a big but reasonable goal and break that goal into smaller and smaller steps. Look over your goal-setting worksheet from the Starting Out section and step yourself through the process. Make sure that your goal is realistic. Set yourself up for success. Making big changes too fast sets you up for failure. I want you to succeed, so please start small.

You can achieve your goals by maintaining a healthy diet, watching your portions, and exercising. A combination of all three will give you the best results. There are no shortcuts. The sooner you begin, the more motivated you will stay because you will start to see changes. It is very empowering to see the results of your hard work.

Continue to retest yourself throughout the program. I teach weekly exercise classes to groups of women, and the results these women see from just that one workout a week are amazing. Keep checking in with yourself to make sure your progress is moving in the direction you want. If you are not seeing the results you want, review your goals, make sure they are realistic, be honest about the commitment you have made, and give your body enough time to make the changes you want.

Warming Up

Whether you're weight training, cardio training, or working on your flexibility, every workout session needs to begin with a warm-up period. This is a critical yet basic component of each workout session. Don't skip it. The warm-up allows your body 5–10 minutes to get ready for the remainder of the workout. By easing your body into your workouts, you allow time for an adjustment period both physically and mentally. Your muscles start to get more blood flow, your brain starts to adjust to the workout mode of the day, and you protect your body from injury by spending these critical minutes in transition.

Here is a five-minute warm-up sequence you can do anywhere. If you don't like this warm-up, just walk moderately on a sidewalk or on a treadmill, or cycle slowly on an outdoor bike or an exercise bike . . . you get the idea. Ease into your workout and warm your body before moving into the heart of your workout. This warm-up sequence is for any workout.

General Rules for Resistance Training

• Always breathe! Holding your breath can send your blood pressure through the ceiling.

• Don't do it if it hurts.

• Perfect form is required. If you feel like you can't achieve perfect form, hire a trainer to assist you.

• Move slowly and in a controlled manner, using approximately a 4/3 count. (That is, count to four while moving in/up/out, and then count to three while moving out/down/in.)

• Increase the amount of resistance when your current level no longer challenges you.

• Move through the progression outlined in this book for best results.

Five-minute Warm-up

1. Slow march in place for 30 seconds.

2. March out/out in/in for 30 seconds.

3. Scissor for 30 seconds.

4. Half jack for 30 seconds.

5. Step touch for 30 seconds.

6. Repeat sequence.

Slow march in place. This is self-explanatory.

March out/out in/in. Continue to march steadily, but now move your legs to a wide stance; move your feet from shoulder width to wider than shoulder width. Then return them back to shoulder width stance, and repeat.

Scissor. Swing your arms straight up and in front of you, stopping at ear level; then bring them back down. As you do this, step your right foot behind you; then move it forward to normal stance. Repeat with your left foot. Time your arm movements so that they go up as a foot steps back, and so that your arms come down when a foot steps forward to normal stance.

Half jack. Step out with your right leg to your right side as your right arm moves up toward your face. Bring your right arm back down as you step in with your right leg. Then step out with your left foot to your left side, while your left arm moves up toward your face. Bring your left arm back down as you step in with your left leg. Make sure your feet do not leave the floor. Repeat the sequence.

Step touch. Step your left foot to the left, then bring your right foot next to your left foot. Follow this by stepping your right foot to the right and bringing left foot next to your right foot. Repeat the sequence.

A Word on the Strength Exercises

The program I have designed for you is meant to be functional, meaning all exercises replicate real-life movement. I believe health, rather than looking good, is the actual reason most brides want to get fit—having nice arm muscles that show on your wedding day is simply the by-product of your fitness routine. By using exercises that replicate real-life movement, you are preparing yourself for the moves you will do day in and day out for the rest of your life. The exercises are easy to do and learn, and they require very little equipment. They are also very effective in building muscular strength and endurance, and for giving you a "toned" look.

Some Basic Rules

Strength training two times per week is a good place to begin. To do so, follow the routine for Level One. Use weights or bands that allow you to perform 8–12 repetitions with perfect form. Do two sets per exercise using enough resistance so that you feel fatigued by the end of the second set. Make sure you warm up prior to using the weights. To make sure your muscles are warm, do a 5–10 minute warm-up, as described in the previous section.

Make sure you take a day off between working your muscle groups. If you are doing the full body workout outlined in Chapter 8, you will be skipping at least one day between weight-training sessions. Your muscles need a day to recover. If you feel awkward doing the exercises or are having trouble with the movements, find a workout buddy to watch and correct you. In addition, doing the exercises in front of a mirror will help you maintain good form. Throughout the program, I have also included tips and common errors you can consult to check that you are performing the exercises properly.

If you don't feel like you are "getting" a particular exercise, you may want to spend the money to hire a personal trainer for a couple of lessons to teach you proper form. The routine I have designed is meant to be very easy, but everyone has a different level of coordination and mind/body connection. And the last thing I want is for you to get injured.

I have developed three weight routines for you and have recommended when to move from Level One to Level Two and then to Level Three. These are only recommendations. If you are finding Level One too easy for you before 12 weeks, go ahead and move to Level Two. Feel free to mix and match within the routines, keeping the exercises you like and dropping those you don't particularly care for. It is important you continue progressing, adding more weight or more reps to improve. Remember, don't do it if it hurts! And make sure your form is always perfect and that you are executing these exercises properly. You don't want to have to limp down the aisle or show up with your arm in a sling on your wedding day.

CHAPTER 8

Level One: Setting Your Baseline

This chapter includes:
- Workout Schedule for Weeks 1–6

Specific exercise descriptions for Level One:

Half Squats with a Ball Against the Wall	Overhead Press, Seated
Inner and Outer Thigh Exercise	Bicep Curls Alternating Sides
Supine Bridge	Tricep Extensions Alternating Sides
Chest Press with Bands	TVA Holds
Standing Rows with Bands	Abdominal Crunch on the Ball
Push-ups	Bicycle Maneuver
	Back Extensions on Floor

Stretching routine:

Neck	Hip
Shoulders and arms	Quadriceps
Sides	Inner thighs
Chest	Runner stretch
Upper back	Triceps
Hamstring	Back

Workout Schedule for Weeks 1–6

Here is a weekly schedule to help get you going on your fitness program. Schedule the time in your daily planner just like any other appointment you make. Keep this appointment; it's important! If you are just beginning to exercise on a regular basis, you should start at this first level. Don't jump ahead because you are running out of time or your wedding day is getting closer. Just as you had to date before getting married, you have to invest some time in exercising to get long-term results. Start slow, build a good base, and then grow from that base. Not only will this attitude work with your marriage, it also will work with your exercise program.

Week 1

Cardio: Do two sessions this week. Work at an RPE of 4–6 for up to 30 minutes. Use any type of cardio workout you like. (See Modes of Cardiorespiratory Exercise on page 53 for types of cardio programs you can try.)

WEEK	Mon	Tues	Wed	Thurs	Fri	Sat	Sun
1	Cardio 30 RPE 4–6	Off	Weights	Cardio 30 RPE 4–6	Off	Weights	Off
2	Cardio 30 RPE 4–6	Off	Weights	Cardio 30 RPE 4–6	Off	Weights	Off
3	Off	Cardio 30 RPE 4–6	Weights	Cardio 30 RPE 4–6	Off	Weights	Off
4	Cardio 30 RPE 4–6	Off	Weights	Cardio 30 RPE 4–6	Off	Weights	Off
5	Cardio 30–35 RPE 5–7	Off	Weights	Cardio 30–35 RPE 5–7	Off	Weights	Off
6	Cardio 35 RPE 5–7	Off	Weights	Cardio 35 RPE 5–7	Off	Weights	Off

Whatever workout you choose, make sure it is an activity you will enjoy doing. If you decide to work out in a gym, feel free to break up the time using different machines in the room. For example, you could use the treadmill for five minutes, then move to the stationary bike for five minutes, then move to the elliptical machine for five minutes. Make sure you count only the minutes you are working out and not the time in between routines. I recommend multiple routines because it will break up the monotony. In addition, using multiple routines gives your body a well-rounded program that stresses it in many ways rather than stressing it in the same way over and over again. This will help you prevent injury and make your time exercising as effective as possible.

Strength training: Do two sessions this week, with 8–12 reps per set. At this early stage, just do two sets. We will work up to three sets later in the program.

Flexibility: After every cardio and strength-training session, stretch for 6–10 minutes.

Week 2

Cardio: Do two sessions this week. Work at an RPE of 4–6 for up to 30 minutes. Use any type of exercise you like because you are still just getting started. While working out, you should be able to talk and you should feel like you can sustain the exercise for the full time you've allotted. If you can't make the full 30 minutes, that's OK. *Do only what you can.* Don't kill yourself. Instead, work at a level that's enjoyable but where you know you are working your body. Give yourself time to work up to the full 30 minutes.

Strength training: Do two sessions this week, with 8–12 reps per set and two sets of each exercise.

Flexibility: After every cardio and strength-training session, stretch for 6–10 minutes.

Week 3

Cardio: Do two sessions this week. Work at an RPE of 4–6 for up to 30 minutes.

Strength training: Do two sessions this week, with 8–12 reps per set. At this point, if you have been doing only 8 reps per set, begin working toward 10 reps per set and two sets of each exercise.

Flexibility: After every cardio and strength-training session, stretch for 6–10 minutes.

Week 4

Cardio: Do two sessions this week. Work at an RPE of 4–6 for up to 30 minutes. Remember to mix it up. You want to keep stressing your system, and it's easiest if you are creating stress in a variety of ways.

Strength training: Do two sessions this week. Continue working toward 10–12 reps per set with perfect form and two sets of each exercise.

Flexibility: After every cardio and strength-training session, stretch for 6–10 minutes.

Week 5

Cardio: Do two sessions this week. Increase your workout to an RPE of 5–7 for 30–35 minutes.

Strength training: Do two sessions this week, aiming for 10–12 reps per set and two sets of each exercise. If any of the exercises are getting easy for you, add either weight or resistance (but only if your form is perfect) or reps. The way to determine that it is time to add more weight/resistance is when you can easily perform 12 reps per set with perfect form. At this point increase the weight (5–10%), add reps (up to 15 per set), or add sets (1). The goal is to stress your muscles. If you are not stressing them, they will not change.

Flexibility: After every cardio and strength-training session, stretch for 6–10 minutes.

Week 6

Cardio: Do two sessions this week. Work at an RPE of 5–7 for 30–35 minutes.

Strength training: Do two sessions this week, aiming for 12 reps per set and two sets of each exercise.

Flexibility: After every cardio and strength-training session, stretch for 6–10 minutes.

After Week 6, if you have reached a point where 30-35 minutes of cardio activity is fairly easy for you, go ahead and move to Level Two, Week 7 (see page 78). If not, stay at this level until you feel comfortable and confident that it's time to move forward. (Reminder: Before moving on to Level Two, remember to perform the fitness tests outlined in Chapter 6 and record your scores again.)

Cardiovascular Training for Levels One, Two, and Three

What is cardiorespiratory fitness? According to the American College of Sports Medicine, "It is the improvement in the ability of the heart to deliver oxygen to the working muscles and is the muscles' ability to generate energy with oxygen resulting in increased endurance performance. Improvement in cardiorespiratory fitness is measured by assessing the change in VO2max [your body's ability to utilize oxygen in the blood], which is directly related to the frequency, duration, and intensity of exercise."

Modes of Cardiorespiratory Exercise

Inside: Most gyms have a room full of cardio equipment. Treadmills, step machines, stationary bicycles, and rowing machines are all meant to give you a cardio workout. The way these machines succeed in doing this is by working your large muscle groups over prolonged periods of time; these activities are also rhythmic and aerobic in nature. Swimming, dancing, and rope skipping are other non-machine-based indoor cardio exercises. Most gyms also offer group fitness classes. Bench step and aerobics classes are good choices for a cardio workout for those who enjoy working out in groups.

Outside: Walking, running, biking, hiking, rowing a boat, cross-country skiing, swimming, and climbing mountains—these are all great outdoor cardio-based exercises.

The key to finding the right cardio exercise for you is in doing what you like, at a level you can maintain for increasing periods of time. Start slowly and progress slowly. Listen to your body, and if the activity causes pain, choose something else.

Half Squats with a Ball Against the Wall
(Works Leg and Gluteal Muscles)

USING THE WALL takes some of your body weight off your frame, which allows you to work up to a full squat slowly. You will use all your major leg muscles with this exercise.

1. Stand facing away from the wall.

2. Place the ball behind you, approximately at the curve of your lower back.

3. Your feet should be roughly 12 inches in front of your body and a comfortable distance apart. Start with your feet 12 inches or shoulder width apart, facing away from the wall. Adjust your stance to a comfort point.

4. Leaning into the ball, slowly lower yourself toward the floor, bending your knees as you go. As you lower yourself, the ball should roll up your back.

5. Be sure your weight is over your whole foot, not over your toes. If your toes are taking the brunt of the weight, move your feet further in front of your body, away from the wall. (At all stages of this exercise, you should be able to see your toes.)

6. Keep your chest and eyes up.

7. Lower yourself until your thighs are parallel to the floor. If you are new to this exercise, it may take some time to reach this depth. If so, just lower yourself to a point that feels right for you to be able to do 8–10 reps of this exercise. Then in subsequent sessions, work on lowering yourself further each time, until your thighs are parallel to the floor.

8. Move back to the start position.

9. Repeat.

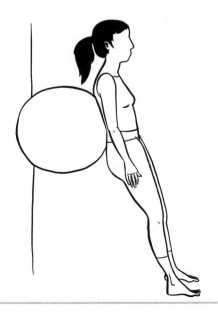
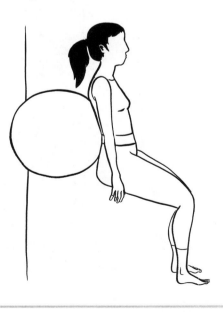

Inner and Outer Thigh Exercise
(Works Inner and Outer Thighs)

THIS EXERCISE WORKS your abductors (outer thighs) and adductors (inner thighs):

1. Lie on your back, legs straight up, with soles of your feet facing the ceiling.

2. Place your arms out at your sides. They should be at a 45-degree angle from your hips.

3. Keep your head on the floor at all times.

4. While inhaling, open your legs to either side and extend them out as far as feels comfortable.

5. While exhaling, close your legs.

6. Repeat.

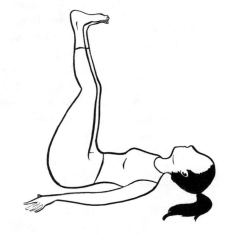

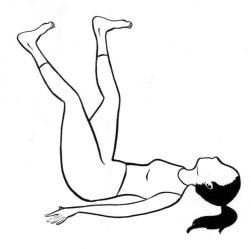

Supine Bridge

(Works Hamstrings, Glutes, Abdominals, and Back)

1. Lie on your back.

2. Bend your knees. Your feet should be flat on the floor, 12–18 inches away from your buttocks.

3. Keep your arms flat on the floor and at your sides throughout this exercise.

4. Keep your head resting on a mat.

5. Lift your hips until your body core (your trunk region) raises up off the floor. Only your shoulders and head should be touching the floor at this point. (Before starting this exercise, you can place a towel under your shoulder blades for extra cushioning.)

6. After lifting your hips as high as you can go, hold the position for 10 seconds, then slowly lower yourself back to the floor.

7. Repeat.

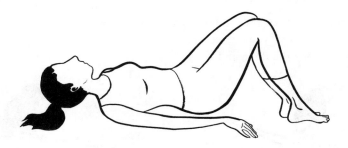

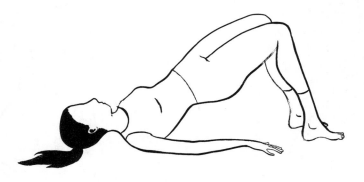

Chest Press with Bands
(Works the Chest Muscles)

1. Attach a resistance band to a door or an object behind you at approximately chest height. (Use a door attachment—a piece of cord/webbing that fits into a door jam; you can purchase one with your resistance band—or put the bands around a stationary object.)

2. With a band handle in each hand, walk away from the attachment point until the band is taut.

3. Keep a staggered stance (one foot in front of the other) to give you more stability. Change the lead foot after each set.

4. Stand up straight and keep your abdominal muscles tight. Hold your chest up, have your palms face the floor, and keep your elbows at a 90-degree angle at chest height.

5. Move the handles of the bands forward in a steady pushing motion while keeping your wrists straight.

6. Press to the end of your range of motion or until your hands meet in front of you at chest level. You may need to adjust your distance from the attachment point so that your arms can go through the full range of motion.

7. Release the push, and return backward through these steps until you reach your starting point.

8. Repeat.

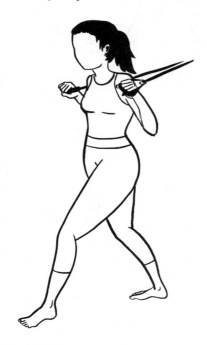
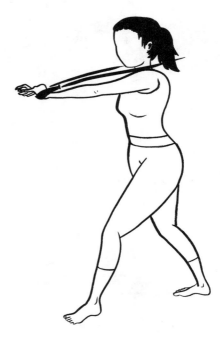

Standing Rows with Bands
(Works the Upper Back)

THIS EXERCISE IS GREAT for posture. It helps improve your upper back muscles, your ability to balance, and your stability all at once.

1. Secure the resistance band at a chest-high attachment point.

2. Face the attachment point, standing far enough away that the band is taut.

3. Take the band handles in your hands, keeping your wrists straight, palms facing each other. Do not shrug your shoulders. Keep your shoulder blades down.

4. At all times, your feet should be shoulder width apart, with your knees slightly bent. Bend your knees enough to keep a solid stance. Pull the band toward you, keeping your elbows at your side, so they brush your torso when you are pulling in and moving your hands toward your chest. The movement should be slow and steady.

5. Release at the same speed you pulled the band toward you, back to the full extended position.

6. Repeat.

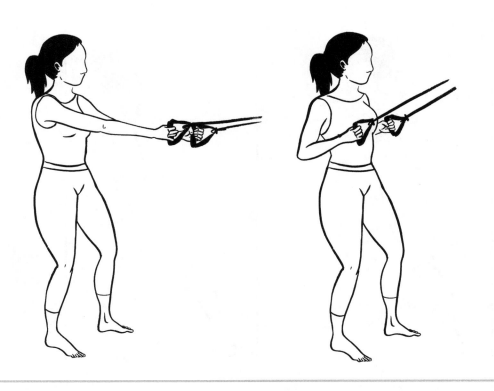

Push-up Variation # 1: Wall Push-ups
(Works Shoulders, Chest, and Abs)

I LOVE PUSH-UPS. The great thing about them is they work a number of major muscle groups. When starting out with push-ups, don't worry about how many you can do; you can continue to work your way to full body push-ups by the end of this program. Here are my three variations to performing a standard push-up.

1. Stand facing a wall. The farther away your feet are from the wall, the harder the push-up will be.

2. Place your palms on the wall, just below your shoulders. Your palms should be a bit farther apart than your shoulders.

3. Keeping your body rigid in a straight line, lean in toward the wall. (You may need to turn your head to your left or your right when at your closest point to the wall.)

4. Return to the start position.

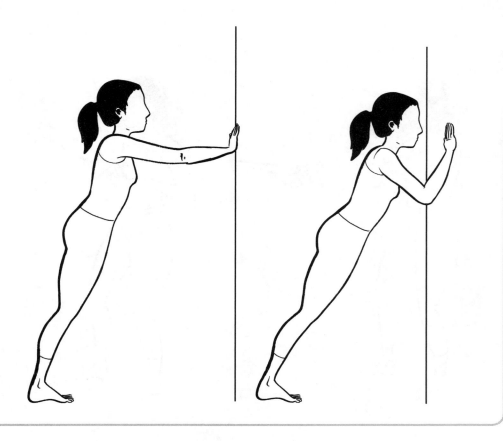

Push-up Variation # 2: Counter Push-ups
(Works Shoulders, Chest, and Abs)

YOU WILL GET A BETTER core workout doing a counter push-up than you will using the ball or your knees. Once the wall push-up feels easy, try the counter push-up and progress lower and lower until you reach the floor. To do this, find a series of ledges of varying height that you can use for your push-ups throughout the Healthy Bride workout program: perhaps a low counter-top to start with, then a bench, then a step, and then eventually, the floor. The lower the ledge, the harder the push-up will be. A very simple, low-tech way to progress to lower ledges is to use a staircase. Stand facing a staircase and place your hands on about the fifth or sixth step. As you get better at push-ups, work your way down the staircase.

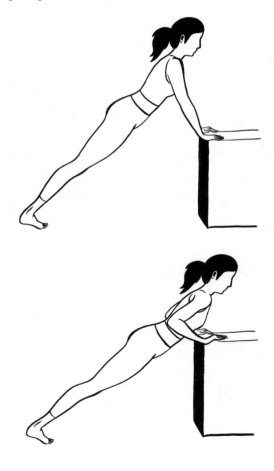

Push-up Variation #3: Push-up Over the Ball
(Works Shoulders, Chest, and Abs)

1. From a standing position, crouch down behind the exercise ball. Place your abdomen on top of the ball and roll forward until your hands reach the ground.

2. Walk out with your hands as far as you feel comfortable.

3. Pull in your abs, and keep your body in a straight line.

4. Keep your shoulders over your elbows and elbows over your wrists.

5. Lower yourself down as far as you feel comfortable. You should be able to get low enough that the part of your arms above your elbows is parallel to the floor.

6. Push back up to the start position.

7. Repeat.

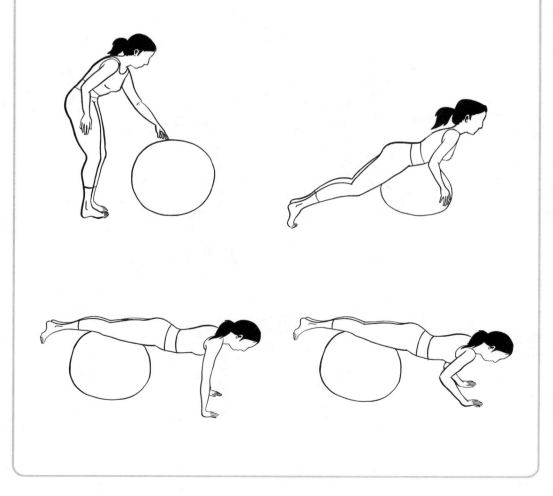

Overhead Press, Seated

(Works Shoulders)

1. Sit in a chair.

2. Place a resistance band under the seat of the chair, or sit on the band while seated.

3. Grab the left side of the band in your left hand and the right side of the band in your right hand. Hold your palms facing forward.

4. Push the band up, straightening your arms, while bringing your hands together over your head.

5. Whenever your arms are over your head, be sure you can see your elbows in your peripheral vision. This helps shield you from possible shoulder injury.

6. Lower the band back to the start position.

7. Repeat.

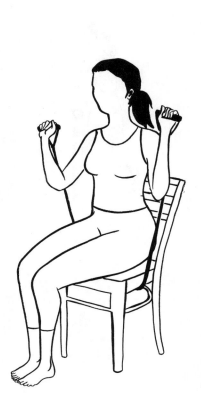 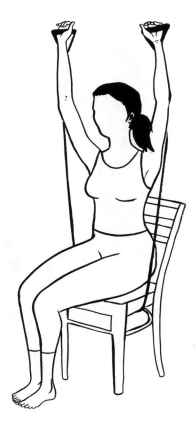

Bicep Curls Alternating Sides
(Works Biceps)

1. Stand with your feet shoulder width apart and your knees slightly bent.

2. If using a resistance band, stand on the band with one foot. As an alternative, you can use dumbbells.

3. Hold one dumbbell or one band handle in each hand. Keep your hands at your sides, palms facing forward.

4. Curl one arm up toward your shoulder, moving the arm only from your elbow.

Make sure you do not move your shoulder joint. At the "top" of the curl (the end of your range of motion), your palm should be facing your bicep.

5. Lower that arm back to the start position.

6. Curl the second arm exactly as you did the first arm.

7. Lower that arm back to start position.

8. Repeat.

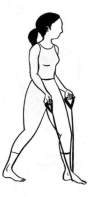
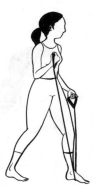
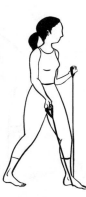

Tricep Extensions Alternating Sides
(Works Triceps)

1. Stand with your feet shoulder width apart and your knees slightly bent.

2. Using one hand, grip one handle of the resistance band behind your head. With your other hand, grasp the other end of the elastic band behind your back at the level most comfortable for you. (Refer to the following illustration.)

3. Keep your lower hand stationary at your back, and extend your higher hand over your head.

4. Keep your upper elbow pointed up at all times; do not drop it toward your side.

5. Extend your top arm up. Be careful not to move from your shoulder; move only at your elbow.

6. Slowly lower the top arm and repeat.

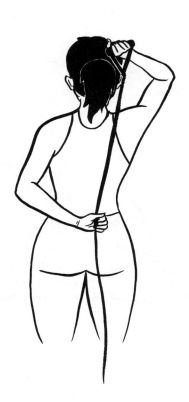
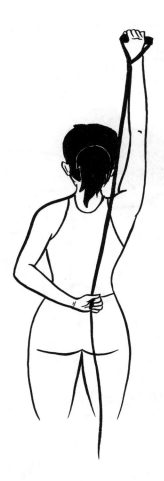

TVA Holds
(Works Transverse Abdominal Muscles)

TO WORK YOUR BODY'S CORE, first engage your deepest abdominal muscles by coughing once. The muscle you feel contracting deep in your abdomen is your *transverse abdominis.* This exercise should precede your other abdominal work. Note that the movements you make during this exercise will be very small.

1. Get on the floor on all fours. Your hands and knees should be on the floor. The space between your hands should be as wide as the space between your knees, and your back should be flat. Pull your belly button toward your spine and hold for a count of three.

2. Repeat up to 10 times.

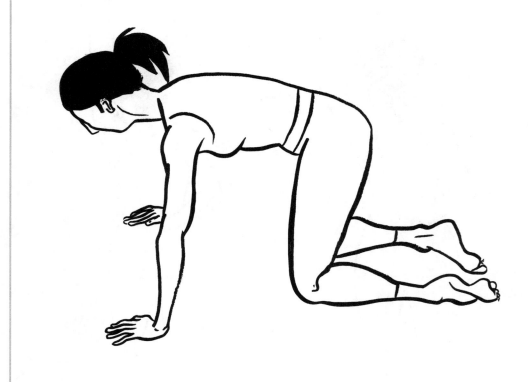

Abdominal Crunches on Ball

(Works Abs and Neck)

THIS IS THE BEST abdominal workout around. Before you start this exercise, be sure you are comfortable and stable on the ball. Do this by sitting on the ball. Then bounce up and down on the ball. Follow that by swiveling your hips on the ball. If you feel OK, proceed. If not, start by doing your crunches on the floor and work up to doing them on the ball by following these steps:

1. Sit on top of the ball and slowly walk your feet forward, away from the ball, until your lower back is supported on the ball. When you begin this exercise, you may drop your hips closer to the floor. This relieves your neck and abs of some of the work and engages your quads to do more of the work.

2. Your hands can be either on your thighs, crossed at your chest, or with your fingers touching your temples. Do not cradle your head in your hands; you need to build strong neck muscles too, and this exercise will help you do so.

3. Lay back over the ball, face up, with your back matching the curvature of the ball. *This is your starting position.*

4. Draw your navel toward your spine, and "crunch" (or roll) your shoulders toward your hips. (This is a small movement that creates a 30- to 45-degree angle of space between your back and the ball.)

5. Be sure to keep your neck in its neutral position. Your chin should not be tucked, but in a straight line from your shoulders to the top of your head.

6. Lower yourself back to the starting position.

7. Repeat the crunches.

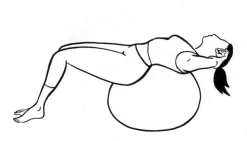 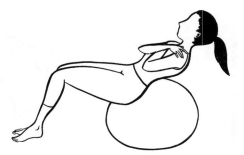

Bicycle Maneuver
(Works Abdominal Oblique Muscles)

1. Lie flat on the floor with your lower back pressed to the ground.

2. Put your hands on top of your shoulders (elbows point out, not forward).

3. Bring your knees up to about a 45-degree angle and rotate your legs as if they were pedaling a bicycle.

4. Keep rotating your legs as you bring your left elbow to your right knee, and then your right elbow to your left knee.

5. Breathe evenly as you continue the exercise.

6. Perform 8–12 reps on each side, or go until you feel fatigued.

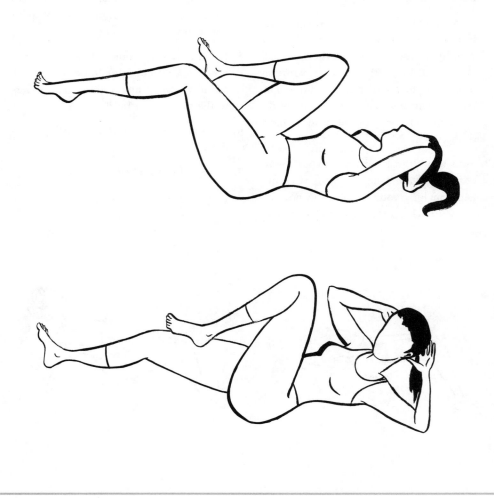

Back Extensions on Floor
(Works the Lower Back)

1. Lie flat on the floor, face down.

2. Place your arms straight above your head, keeping them flat against the floor.

3. Raise your right arm and left leg at the same time, coming up as high as you feel comfortable.

4. Hold for a count of three, then lower your arm and leg.

5. Raise your left arm and right leg at the same time, coming up as high as you feel comfortable.

6. Hold for a count of three, then lower both.

7. Repeat.

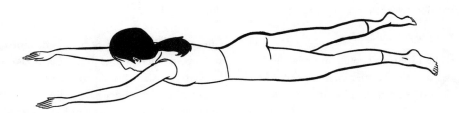

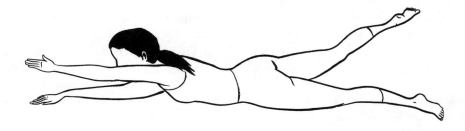

Flexibility Training

(for Levels One, Two, and Three)

TO IMPROVE FLEXIBILITY, it is important to stretch all major muscle groups you worked during your exercise sessions. Follow this stretching routine after each exercise session, both cardio and resistance. This routine should feel really good. Use the illustrations as your guide, and do the best you can. Some general rules for stretching include:

- Hold the stretch to the point of minor discomfort (feeling a pull) for 30–60 seconds.

- If the stretch hurts, don't do it.

- Do not bounce!

- The idea is to stretch and relax at the same time. Remember, this should feel good—not painful or uncomfortable.

Many ways to stretch a muscle group exist. The following stretches are only suggestions. Feel free to add your own favorite stretches to the routine; just make sure they are safe.

Neck. Slowly drop your neck forward, and then roll it from shoulder to shoulder. When it feels loosened up, roll your head in a full circle. Be careful not to roll back too far. Don't strain.

Shoulders and arms. Stand near a wall or doorway. Face the wall and stretch your left arm out. Hold onto the doorway or press against the wall with your left hand open, thumb pointing toward the ceiling, hand at shoulder height. Slowly turn away from the arm against the wall or doorway, with your head facing to the right. Keep your hips straight ahead. Repeat with your right arm, turning your head to the left to perform the stretch.

Sides. Stand with feet shoulder width apart and your knees slightly bent. Put your left hand on left hip, and bend sideways at your waist, to your left. Repeat with your right hand on your right hip, bending to the right. For a more challenging stretch, put both arms overhead while you bend to one side, then the other.

Chest. Stand in front of an open doorway, with your back to the door frame. Reach behind you with both hands and grasp the door frame at shoulder height. Let your arms straighten behind you as you lean forward.

Upper back. Lace your fingers together and face your palms away from you. Reach your arms forward, pushing your hands away in front of you, while rounding your back.

Hamstring. Place one foot on a step, chair, bench, or ball—nothing too high. Keep the leg on the floor slightly bent, while keeping the outstretched leg on the ledge straight. Look ahead and bend forward at the waist until you feel the stretch in the back of your leg. Repeat on both legs.

Hip. Sit on the floor holding your right leg straight in front of you. Bend your left leg, cross your left foot over your right leg, and rest your left foot to the outside of your

Flexibility Training
(for Levels One, Two, and Three)

right knee. Pull your left knee across your body toward your right shoulder until you feel an easy stretch in your hip. Hold, then repeat on the opposite side.

Quadriceps. To do this stretch, you might want to stand in front of a wall for balance. Fold your right leg behind you so that your right foot meets your buttocks (or comes as close as you can to your buttocks). Hold the top of your right foot with your left hand and gently pull your heel further toward your buttocks. Hold. Make sure your knee is pointing straight down, toward the floor. Repeat using your right hand and left leg.

Inner thighs. In a sitting position, bring the soles of your feet together (knees should be bent) and hold them with your hands. Gently lower your chest to the floor, feeling the stretch in your groin and inner thigh area.

Runner stretch. From a standing position, take a huge step forward with your left leg. Take as big a step forward as possible, bending your left knee, and keeping your right leg straight with your toes on the floor. Bend your left knee until it is directly above your left ankle. Your right knee should now be touching the floor. Place your hands flat against the floor, on each side of your left foot. Bend further forward, lowering your hips downward, and feel the stretch in the hip flexor muscles (from the front of your hips down to your thighs). Repeat, switching leg positions.

Triceps. With your arms over your head, grab your left elbow with your right hand. Gently pull the elbow behind your head and lower your left hand down your back between your shoulder blades. Feel the stretch. Repeat, using opposite hands and elbow.

Back. I've included two stretches here for your back:
• *Cat stretch:* Get on all fours on the floor (hands and knees touching the floor). Round your back as though you are laying over a beach ball, lowering your head while you do so. Now arch your back and bring your head up. Repeat.
• *Lower-back stretch:* On all fours (hands and knees touching the floor), thread your right hand between your left shoulder and left knee, lowering your right shoulder all the way to the floor. Keep your right arm straight and flat against the floor. Return to the starting position and repeat on the opposite side.

Neck Stretch

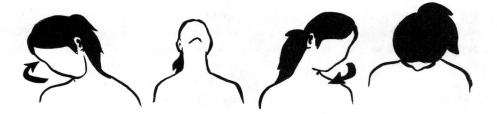

Shoulders and Arms

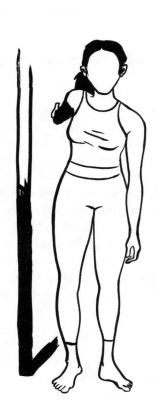
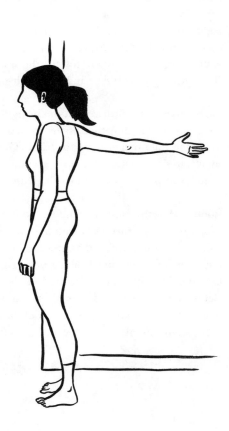

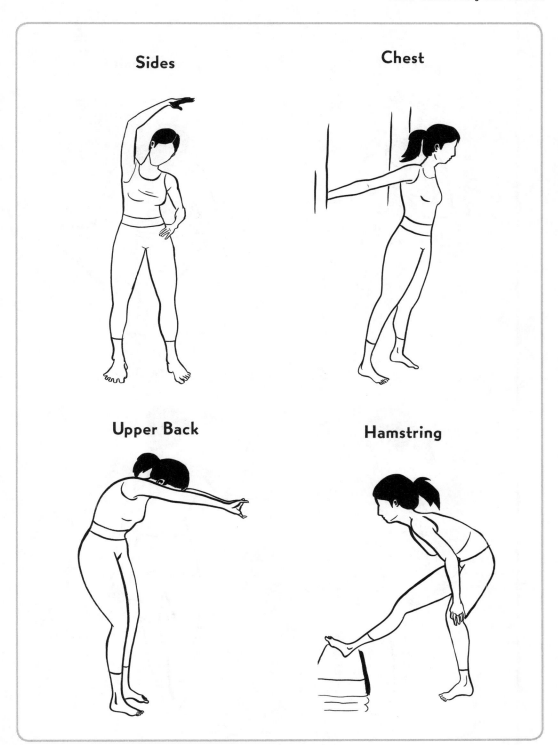

Sides

Chest

Upper Back

Hamstring

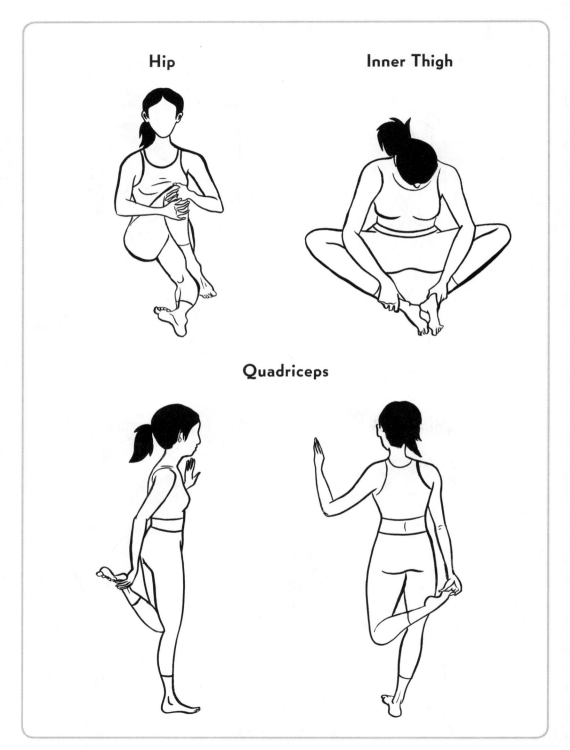

Hip

Inner Thigh

Quadriceps

Runner Stretch

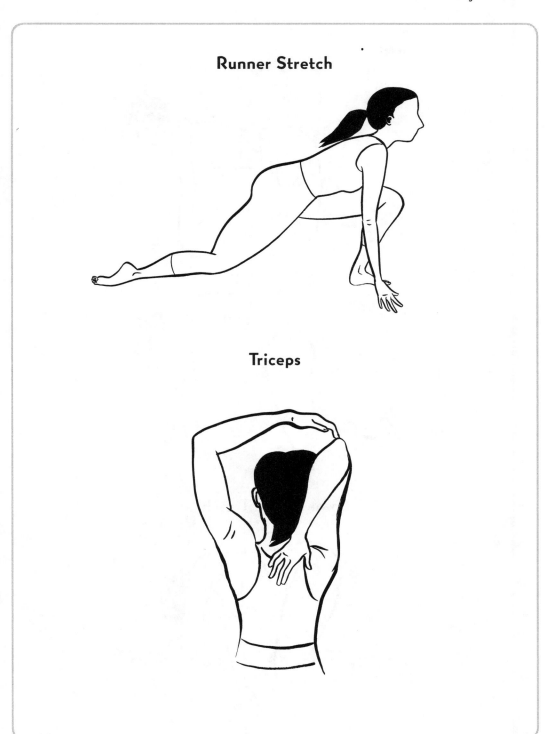

Triceps

Cat Stretch

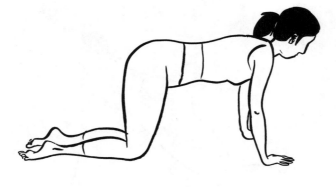

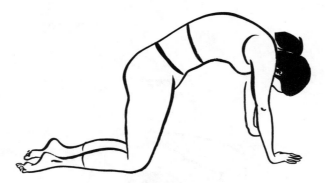

Lower-back Stretch

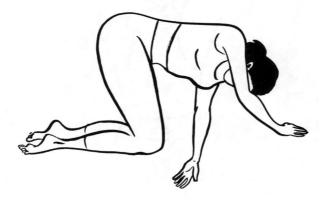

CHAPTER 9

Level Two: Improvement Stage

Congratulations! You have now established a good base and are ready to move forward to the next level of this program. Continue progressing toward your health and fitness goals. Perform the fitness tests outlined in Chapter 6 now and record your progress. Compare these scores to your last set and celebrate your improvement!

During this improvement phase, we will increase one FITT principle at a time. This means increasing frequency, intensity, and time to continue progressively overloading your system enough to get it to change. It is important to increase only one factor at a time in this phase. The goal is to continue to move you forward at a rate your body can manage. If you get injured, your progress will stop or be delayed, which you certainly don't want to happen.

Watch out for red flags during this stage, such as dreading the workout because it's getting too long or too hard, or because it hurts. These are all indications that you are doing too much; in such cases, scale your routine back to a level you are more comfortable with.

During this stage, we will increase your workout by about 10 percent a week. For the next few weeks, we will start by increasing time.

Weeks 7–12: Part One of Improvement

This section includes:

• Revised workout schedule

Here is your new schedule for this first part of Level Two. For resistance training, continue with the same exercises you used in Level One.

Workout Schedule for Weeks 7–12

WEEK	Mon	Tues	Wed	Thurs	Fri	Sat	Sun
7	Cardio 35 RPE 5–7	Off	Weights	Cardio 35 RPE 5–7	Off	Weights	Off
8	Cardio 55 RPE 5–7	Off	Weights	Cardio 38 RPE 5–7	Off	Weights	Off
9	Off	Cardio 42 RPE 5–7	Weights	Cardio 42 RPE 5–7	Off	Weights	Off
10	Cardio 45 RPE 5–7	Off	Weights	Cardio 45 RPE 5–7	Off	Weights	Off
11	Cardio 50 RPE 5–7	Off	Weights	Cardio 50 RPE 5–7	Off	Weights	Off
12	Cardio 55 RPE 5–7	Off	Weights	Cardio 55 RPE 5–7	Off	Weights	Off

Week 7

Cardio: Do two sessions this week. Work at an RPE of 5–7 for 35 minutes.

Strength training: Do two sessions this week, aiming for 10–12 reps per set, performing two or three sets. By this week, you can determine when you are ready to add a third set of resistance exercises by following these guidelines: Make sure your form is perfect at two sets before aiming for a third. You may need to use slightly lighter weights to do the third set with perfect form. Make sure you have enough time to do all three sets. If you feel you just don't have the time to add a third set, keep increasing the weight so that you feel fatigued with two sets.

Flexibility: After every cardio and strength-training session, stretch for 6–10 minutes.

Week 8

Cardio: Do two sessions this week. Work at an RPE of 5–7 for 38 minutes.

Strength training: Do two sessions this week, aiming for 10–12 reps per set, performing two or three sets.

Flexibility: After every cardio and strength-training session, stretch for 6–10 minutes.

Week 9

Cardio: Do two sessions this week. Work at an RPE of 5–7 for 42 minutes.

Strength training: Do two sessions this week, aiming for 10–12 reps per set.

Flexibility: After every cardio and strength-training session, stretch for 6–10 minutes.

Week 10

Cardio: Do two sessions this week. Work at an RPE of 5–7 for 45 minutes.

Strength training: Do two sessions this week, aiming for 10–12 reps per set and performing two or three sets.

Flexibility: After every cardio and strength-training session, stretch for 6–10 minutes.

Week 11

Cardio: Do two sessions this week. Work at an RPE of 5–7 for 50 minutes.

Strength training: Do two sessions this week, aiming for 10–12 reps per set and performing two or three sets.

Flexibility: After every cardio and strength-training session, stretch for 6–10 minutes.

Week 12

Cardio: Do two sessions this week. Work at an RPE of 5–7 for 55 minutes.

Strength training: Do two sessions this week, aiming for 10–12 reps per set and performing two or three sets.

Flexibility: After every cardio and strength-training session, stretch for 6–10 minutes.

At the end of Week 12, perform the fitness tests once again to check your progress.

Weeks 13–18: Part Two of Improvement

This section includes:

- Revised workout schedule

- Explanation of interval training

New resistance routine with exercise descriptions:

Walking or Standing Lunges

Hip Bridges

Side Leg Lifts with Band

Adductor Ball Squeeze

Rows with Half Squats

Standing Lat Rows Using Dumbbells

Chest Press on Ball with Dumbbells

Seated Shoulder Press with
    Dumbbells or Bar

Bicep Curls with Both Arms Together

Tricep Extensions Alternating Sides

Supine Heel Drop

Russian Twist on Ball

Abdominal Crunches on Ball

Hip Lifts

Workout Schedule for Weeks 13–18

Here is your new schedule for the second part of Level Two. You will start incorporating interval training within your cardio workouts (marked by the letter "I" in the following schedule). In addition, you will start a brand-new resistance-training program with new exercises. We are shaking up your muscles at this point. Because you have had 12 weeks on the same program, your muscles should have adapted to the stress by now and those exercises should

Workout Schedule for Weeks 13–18

WEEK	Mon	Tues	Wed	Thurs	Fri	Sat	Sun
13	Cardio 55 RPE 5–8	Off	Weights	Cardio 45 I RPE 5–9.5	Off	Weights	Off
14	Cardio 55 RPE 5–8	Off	Weights	Cardio 45 I RPE 5–9.5	Off	Weights	Off
15	Off	Cardio 55	Weights	Cardio 45 I RPE 5–9.5	Off	Weights	Off
16	Cardio 55 RPE 5–8	Off	Weights	Cardio 45 I RPE 5–9.5	Off	Weights	Off
17	Cardio 55 RPE 5–8	Off	Weights	Cardio 50 I RPE 5–9.5	Off	Weights	Off
18	Cardio 55 RPE 5–8	Off	Weights	Cardio 50 I RPE 5–9.5	Off	Weights	Off

be easy for you. It's time to make some changes in your resistance-training routine.

As discussed earlier in the book, for your muscles to continue improving, they need to be stressed. This list of exercises contains modifications of some exercises you did before. Plus, I have added some more difficult exercises. Only do what feels right and comfortable, and only do those exercises that you can do with perfect form. If something hurts or if it doesn't feel right to you, don't do it.

Week 13

Cardio: Do two sessions this week. Work at an RPE of 5–8 for 55 minutes for one of the sessions, and add interval training for the second session at an

RPE of 5–9.5 for 45 minutes. Make sure the "regular" cardio sessions are mixed and that you are varying your mode.

Strength training: Do two sessions this week, aiming for 8–12 reps per set and performing two sets of each of the new exercises.

Flexibility: After every cardio and strength-training session, stretch for 6-10 minutes.

Week 14

Cardio: Do two sessions this week. Work at an RPE of 5–8 for 55 minutes for one of the sessions, and add interval training for the second session at an RPE of 5–9.5 for 45 minutes.

Strength training: Do two sessions this week, aiming for 8–12 reps per set and performing two sets of each of the new exercises.

Flexibility: After every cardio and strength-training session, stretch for 6–10 minutes.

Week 15

Cardio: Do two sessions this week. Work at an RPE of 5–8 for 55 minutes for one of the sessions, and add interval training for the second session at an RPE of 5–9.5 for 45 minutes.

Strength training: Do two sessions this week, aiming for 8–12 reps per set and performing two sets of each of the new exercises.

Flexibility: After every cardio and strength-training session, stretch for 6–10 minutes.

Week 16

Cardio: Do two sessions this week. Work at an RPE of 5–8 for 55 minutes for one of the sessions, and add interval training for the second session at an RPE of 5–9.5 for 45 minutes.

Strength training: Do two sessions this week, aiming for 8–12 reps per set and performing two sets of each of the new exercises.

Flexibility: After every cardio and strength-training session, stretch for 6–10 minutes.

Week 17

Cardio: Do two sessions this week. Work at an RPE of 5–8 for 55 minutes for one of the sessions, and add interval training for the second session at an RPE of 5–9.5 for 50 minutes.

Strength training: Do two sessions this week, aiming for 10–12 reps per set and performing two sets of each of the new exercises.

Flexibility: After every cardio and strength-training session, stretch for 6–10 minutes.

Week 18

Cardio: Do two sessions this week. Work at an RPE of 5–8 for 55 minutes for one of the sessions, and add interval training for the second session at an RPE of 5–9.5 for 50 minutes.

Strength training: Do two sessions this week, aiming for 10–12 reps per set and performing two sets of each of the new exercises.

Flexibility: After every cardio and strength-training session, stretch for 6–10 minutes.

Interval Training

Make one cardio session per week an interval cardio session. Here is a minute-by-minute breakdown of what your interval session should look like:

- **Minute 0–10:** Warm up at an RPE level of 4–6.

- **Minute 11–20:** Work at an RPE level of 6–8.

- **Minute 21–26:** Vary this section of your workout by working at an RPE level of 6–8 for 15 seconds, then bumping up your workload to level 8–9.5 for 30 seconds, and finally resuming a level of 6–8 for 15 seconds. Repeat this cycle for five full minutes.

- **Minute 27 to end of session:** Try to incorporate the varied RPE level routine one to three more times during your workout (for a total of 10–20 minutes of your full cardio workout time). So, if your cardio time is 45 minutes, spend 10–20 minutes of that time cycling through your interval training. When not using these intervals, spend the remainder of your time at a 6–8 RPE level.

If you are a runner, a fun way to add intervals is to use the Fartlek (which means "play" in Swedish) method during your run. According to the Fartlek method, you should be setting mini-intervals that allow you to alter the intensity of your workout. So as you are running, look for trees, telephone poles, and corners, and use them as guideposts. Once you reach each guidepost, change the level of your speed and then select another guidepost within sight to use as your next finish point. Mix it up with different speeds.

For example, you may want to start at a steady pace, then switch to a jog, then switch to a sprint, before finally returning to a steady pace. Have fun with this and choose random times to set up challenges for yourself. You can also add other exercises while doing this. For example, find a set of stairs or a hill to run up and down. One of my favorite intervals is do stairs with push-ups. I will do 10 sets of a staircase and then 33 push-ups and repeat that sequence three times.

Why Add Interval Training?

Interval training is important because the harder you work per minute, the more calories you burn. Also, interval training helps you improve your fitness level. For example, if a woman who weighs 130 pounds works at 6 mets for 30 minutes, she will burn 6.2 calories per minute, which means she will burn a total of 186 calories. (A *met* is a metabolic equivalent that offers a way to measure workload based on heat and energy expended. You will find a "met" button on most exercise equipment. If you enter your correct weight into an exercise machine, it will give you an accurate number of calories burned based on this met equation.) If she works at 11 mets for 30 minutes, she will burn 11.4 calories per minute, burning a total of 342 calories. That's three times the number of calories burned in the same amount of time! As you can see, for busy brides like you, interval training can be a great exercise tool.

If you are walking, it is easy to use the hills on your walk for your interval time. You can also add intensity to a walk by using your arms, skipping, hopping, or crouching. Be creative and make your workout fun.

If you are working out in a gym, make sure you rotate through the various machines. Some machines you will like more than others, so try to eliminate the ones you don't like so much. By rotating through various machines, you stress your system in a variety of ways and help keep your body balanced.

The point is not to add more time to your exercise sessions. As stated earlier, I want your workout time to be effective and reasonable—there is no bride I know who has more than an hour in a day to devote to working out.

Also, keep your limits in mind and don't overdo the high-intensity exercises. Yes, by working at a higher intensity rate you may burn twice as many calories in the same amount of time as a normal workout. However, the downside of high-intensity exercise is that you do run a higher risk of injury, so you don't want to work this hard every day.

Walking Lunges
(Works Hamstrings, Quadriceps, and Glutes)

1. From a standing position, take a giant step forward with one leg and land on the heel of your foot.

2. Bend both knees, slowly lowering your hips to the floor.

3. Make sure your front knee is directly over your ankle; you should be able to see your toes at all times.

4. Bend your back knee so that it is near but not touching the floor.

5. Keep your weight distributed over your entire front foot.

6. Push off with your back foot and bring it forward to standing position. Your feet should now be side by side.

7. Continue walking forward in this fashion, switching leg positions. Start at 10 steps per each leg, and increase how many steps you do over time as this exercise becomes easier.

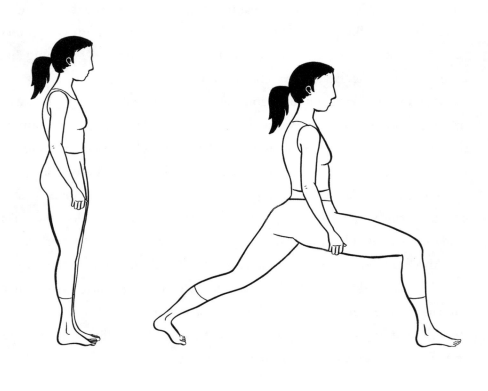

Hip Bridges
(Works the Core, Hips, and Hamstrings)

1. Lie on your back.

2. Bend your knees at a 90-degree angle. Your feet should be flat on the floor and 12–18 inches away from your buttocks.

3. Keep your arms flat on the floor and at your side throughout this exercise.

4. Rest your head on a mat.

5. Lift your hips until your body core (your trunk region) raises up off the floor.

6. Only your shoulders and head should be touching the floor at the top of this exercise. (If you want, you can place a towel under your shoulder blades for extra cushioning.)

7. When your hips reach the highest point they can go, hold the pose for 10 seconds, and then slowly lower yourself back to the floor.

8. Repeat.

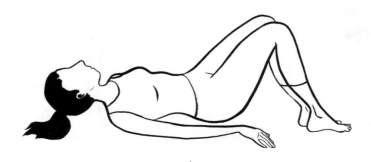

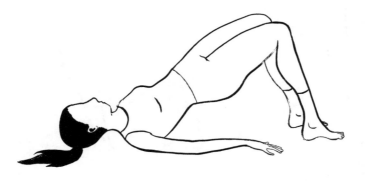

Side Leg Lifts with Band

(Works Outer Thighs, or Abductors)

1. Wrap or tie one resistance band around both of your ankles.

2. Stand next to a wall or chair for balance. You should be perpendicular to the wall or chair so that one leg is closer to it than the other.

3. Slightly bend the leg closest to the wall at your knee.

4. Lift the leg furthest from the wall straight out to the side (away from the wall) and as high as you can go comfortably. This leg can also be slightly bent.

5. Keep your hips forward and your back straight at all times.

6. After completing a set, repeat with the other leg.

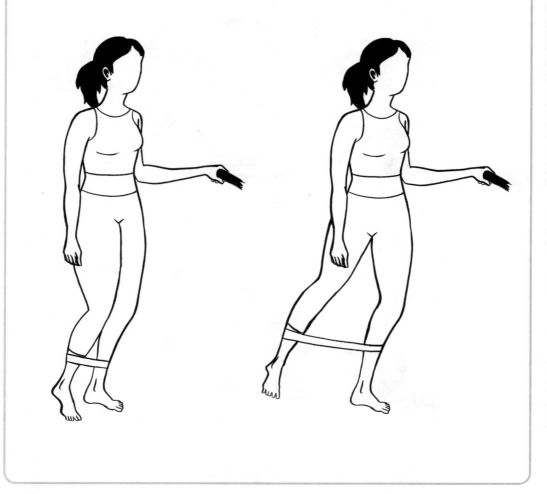

Adductor Ball Squeeze
(Works Inner Thighs, or Adductors)

1. Lie on your back with your legs extended toward the ceiling, knees slightly bent.

2. Place an exercise ball between your legs.

3. Place your arms out to your sides, with your hands positioned out from your hips, hands flat on the floor.

4. Squeeze the ball with your inner thighs.

5. Hold for three to five seconds.

6. Relax and rest one second, then repeat.

7. Do 10 squeezes to start and add more reps as you feel you can.

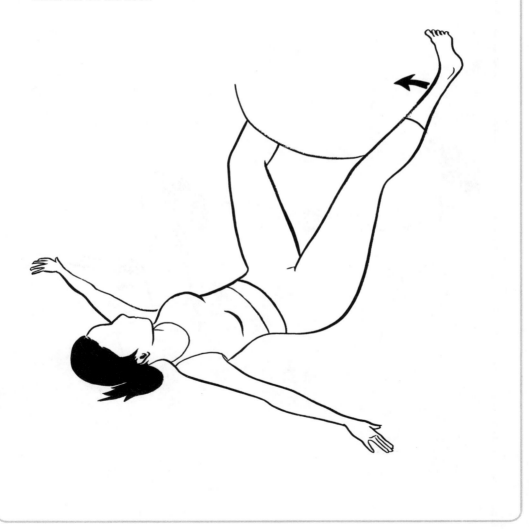

Rows with Half Squats

(Works the Upper Back and Leg Muscles)

1. Follow the directions for Standing Rows with Bands for Level One (see page 59).

2. As you pull your elbows in for your row, add a half squat to the movement. Put your full weight on your heels, sitting back as you squat.

3. Make sure you don't shrug your shoulders during this exercise.

4. Release your arms, and stand back up.

5. Repeat.

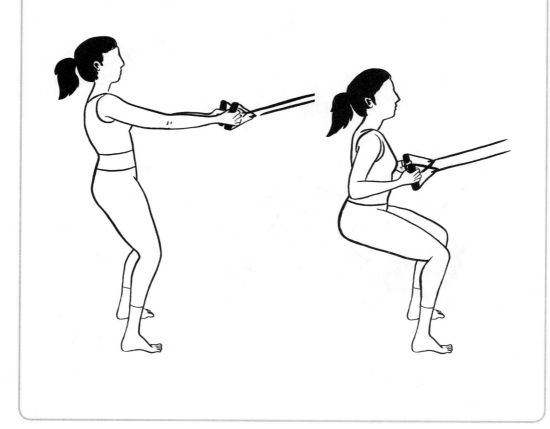

Standing Lat Rows Using Dumbbells
(Works Lats / Back Muscles)

YOUR LATS (latissimus dorsi) are large back muscles that extend, rotate, and lower your arms.

1. In a split stance, with one foot ahead of the other, bend your torso forward so that it's at a 45- to 90-degree angle to the floor.

2. Keep your back flat at all times.

3. Hold a dumbbell in one hand. You can rest your other hand on a chair or the ball if you like.

4. Keeping your abs tucked in, bring your elbow up past your rib cage, finishing with your fist about at your waist.

5. Lower the weight back down.

6. Switch legs with each set.

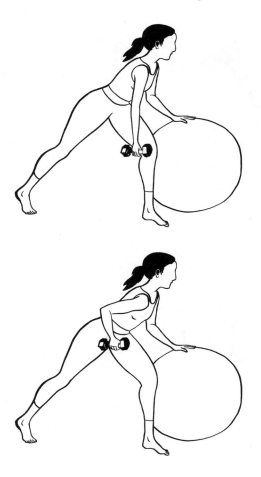

Chest Press on Ball with Dumbbells
(Works Chest and Arms)

1. Lie on the ball with the back of your head and upper back supported on the ball. Hold the dumbbells at your shoulders, next to your chest.

2. Lift your hips up so that your body makes a straight line from your shoulders to your knees (in a bridging fashion).

3. Push the dumbbells straight up above your chest.

4. Lower slowly to the start position. Your upper arms should finish parallel to the floor.

5. Repeat.

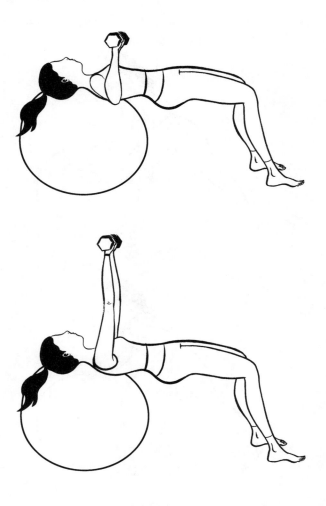

Seated Shoulder Press with Dumbbells

(Works Shoulders and Arms)

1. Sit on the ball holding the dumbbells at shoulder height with palms facing forward.

2. Extend your arms straight up, keeping your elbows in your peripheral vision (slightly ahead of your body).

3. Lower your arms back down to shoulder height.

4. Repeat.

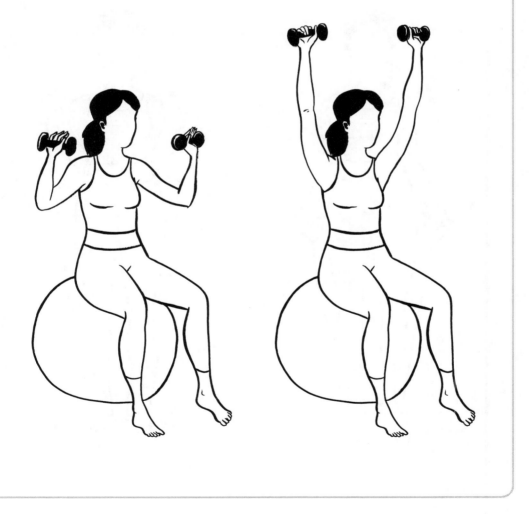

Bicep Curls with Both Arms Together
(Works Biceps)

1. Follow the instructions for Bicep Curls Alternating Sides in Level One (see page 64), but instead of alternating sides, curl both arms at the same time.

2. If you are using a band, stand on the band so that you are holding both handles, one in each hand.

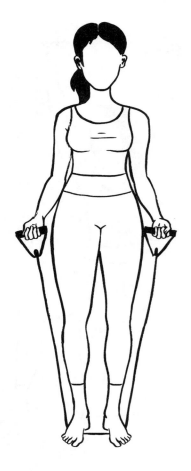
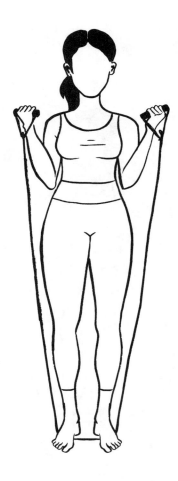

Tricep Extensions Alternating Sides
(Works Triceps)

USE THE SAME EXERCISE performed in Level One (see page 65).

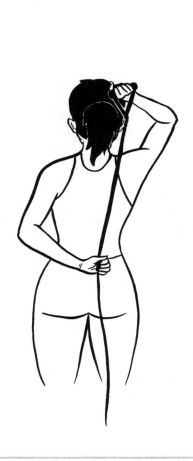 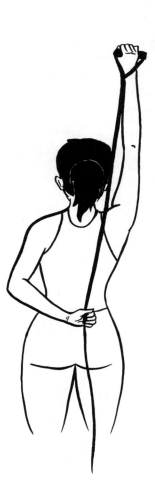

Supine Heel Drop
(Works Inner Abdominal Muscles)

1. Lie on the floor facing up.

2. You should have a natural curve in your lumbar spine, and your head should be resting on the floor. Try placing one hand (palm down) under your lower back and the other hand near your navel (palm down; fingertips pushing in) to feel the muscles at work while holding this neutral position.

3. Bring your knees above your hips, bending your knees so that your shins (and lower legs) are parallel to the floor. Your hips, knees, and ankles should form a 90-degree angle.

4. Slowly lower one foot to the floor, keeping your knee at a 90-degree angle. The other foot remains in the air.

5. As your foot drops, maintain an even pressure on the fingers under your lower back.

6. Before your heel touches the floor and while tightly tucking in your abdominal muscles, bring the lowered leg back up to match your other foot, which should still be in the air.

7. Now repeat the drop sequence with the other leg.

8. Keep your hand under your back to help you maintain consistent abdominal pressure.

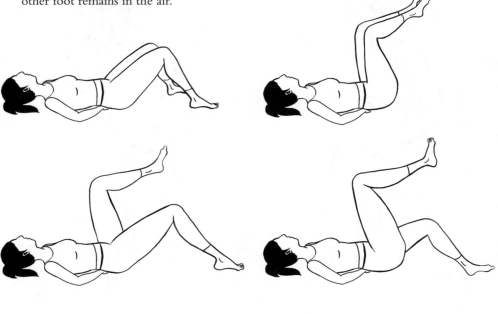

Russian Twist on Ball
(Works Core Area)

1. Sit on top of the ball.

2. Slowly walk your feet forward, away from the ball, until your lower back is supported on the ball.

3. Extend your arms straight up from your chest.

4. Keep your hips parallel to the floor.

5. Rotate your torso all the way to one side. Use your core to initiate the rotation.

6. Roll all the way to the point that your arms are parallel to the floor. Move your head with your arms, keeping your eyes on your hands.

7. Once your arms are parallel to the floor, move back in the opposite direction.

8. Repeat, rotating to the opposite side.

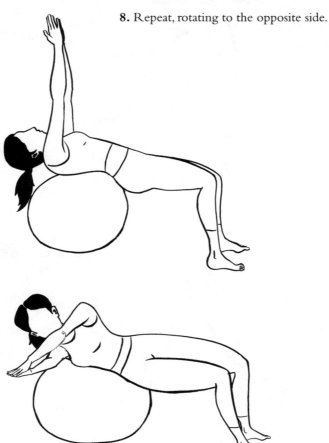

Abdominal Crunches on Ball
(Works Abs and Neck)

USE THE SAME EXERCISE you did in Level One (see page 67). Increase the number of reps per set as the weeks progress.

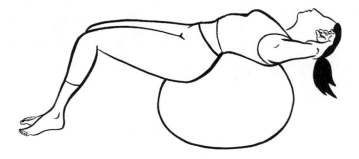

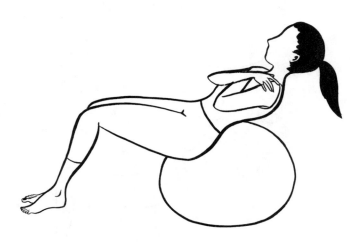

Hip Lifts
(Works Lower Abs)

1. Lie on your back on the floor.

2. Raise your feet in the air, legs straight, until your soles are facing the ceiling and your legs and torso form a 90-degree angle.

3. Extend your arms out to either side of you. They should be flat against the floor.

4. Lift your hips straight up off the ground. Your feet move toward your head. (This should be only a small movement.)

5. Return to start position.

6. Repeat.

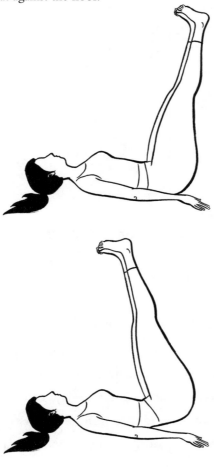

WEEK	Mon	Tues	Wed	Thurs	Fri	Sat	Sun
19	Cardio 55 RPE 5–8	Off	Weights	Cardio 35 I RPE 5-9.5	Cardio Fun	Weights	Off
20	Cardio 55 RPE 5–8	Off	Weights	Cardio 40 I RPE 5-9.5	Off	Weights	Cardio Fun
21	Off	Cardio 55 RPE 5–8	Weights	Cardio 40 I RPE 5-9.5	Cardio Fun	Weights	Off
22	Cardio 55 RPE 5–8	Off	Weights	Cardio 45 I RPE 5-9.5	Off	Weights	Cardio Fun
23	Cardio 55 RPE 5–8	Off	Weights	Cardio 55 I RPE 5-9.5	Cardio Fun	Weights	Off
24	Cardio 55 RPE 5–8	Off	Weights	Cardio 55 I RPE 5-9.5	Cardio Fun	Weights	Off

Weeks 19–24: Part Three of Improvement

This section includes:

• New workout schedule

Workout Schedule for Weeks 19–24

In Part Three of Level Two, you should continue as before, but you also should try to add another day of cardio workout to your weekly schedule. This gives you three days of cardio and two days of weight training per week. You can substitute a day of weight training for an extra day of cardio if you want, but make sure you do not do two consecutive days of weight training.

For your extra cardio day, go do something fun. Go for a hike or a swim, or play a game of basketball, soccer, or tennis—in other words, try something outside your usual routine. Mix it up, and make this activity something you look forward to. For resistance training, keep working on the exercises you used in Part Two of Level Two.

Week 19

Cardio: Do three sessions this week. Work at an RPE of 5–8 for 55 minutes for one of the sessions, and add interval training for the second session at an RPE of 5–9.5 for 35 minutes. Start adding a third, "fun" cardio workout, too. This should be a different activity than you are doing during the other two workouts this week. Make it a hike, bike ride, soccer game, or anything else you enjoy doing outside the normal routine you have developed. Spend a minimum of 35 minutes on this activity, working at any RPE level you wish. Just make it fun.

Strength training: Do two sessions this week, aiming for 10–12 reps per set and performing two or three sets of each exercise. Start with two sets of each exercise and work up to three sets when your body feels ready.

Flexibility: After every cardio and strength-training session, stretch for 6–10 minutes.

Week 20

Cardio: Do three sessions this week. Work at an RPE of 5–8 for 55 minutes for one of the sessions, and add interval training for the second session at an RPE of 5–9.5 for 40 minutes. Spend a minimum of 35 minutes on a third, "fun" cardio session, too.

Strength training: Do two sessions this week, aiming for 10–12 reps per set and performing two or three sets of each exercise.

Flexibility: After every cardio and strength-training session, stretch for 6–10 minutes.

Week 21

Cardio: Do three sessions this week. Work at an RPE of 5-8 for 55 minutes for one of the sessions, and add interval training for the second session at an RPE of 5-9.5 for 40 minutes. Spend a minimum of 35 minutes on a third, "fun" cardio session.

Strength training: Do two sessions this week, aiming for 10-12 reps per set and performing two or three sets of each exercise.

Flexibility: After every cardio and strength-training session, stretch for 6-10 minutes.

Week 22

Cardio: Do three sessions this week. Work at an RPE of 5-8 for 55 minutes or one of the sessions, and add interval training for the second session at an RPE of 5-9.5 for 45 minutes. Spend a minimum of 35 minutes on a third, "fun" cardio session.

Strength training: Do two sessions this week, aiming for 10–12 reps per set and performing two or three sets of each exercise.

Flexibility: After every cardio and strength-training session, stretch for 6–10 minutes.

Week 23

Cardio: Do three sessions this week. Work at an RPE of 5–8 for 55 minutes for one of the sessions, and add interval training for the second session at an RPE of 5–9.5 for 50 minutes. Spend a minimum of 35 minutes on a third, "fun" cardio session.

Strength training: Do two sessions this week, aiming for 10–12 reps per set and performing two or three sets of each exercise.

Flexibility: After every cardio and strength-training session, stretch for 6–10 minutes.

Week 24

Cardio: Do three sessions this week. Work at an RPE of 5–8 for 55 minutes for one of the sessions, and add interval training for the second session at an RPE of 5–9.5 for 55 minutes. Spend a minimum of 35 minutes on a third, "fun" cardio session.

Strength training: Do two sessions this week, aiming for 10–12 reps per set and performing two or three sets of each exercise.

Flexibility: After every cardio and strength-training session, stretch for 6–10 minutes.

Perform fitness tests again at the end of Week 24.

CHAPTER 10

Level Three: Maintenance

Congratulations! I sincerely hope that you are celebrating your victory of sticking to your exercise program this long. You have kept your vows and are ready to develop your own schedule for the program you've found works best for you. By now you might be married. And if you've already gone on your honeymoon, I suspect you were able to swing on the vine into the lovely pool with the waterfall. In addition, you probably feel really healthy, vibrant, and alive. Great job!

This section includes:

- New goal-setting assignment

- New workout schedule (by your own design)

New resistance routine with exercise descriptions:

Full Squats

Walking Lunges with Dumbbells

Hamstring Curls with Ball

Jackknife on Ball

Adductor Ball Squeeze

Side Leg Lifts with Band

Lying Dumbbell Fly and Pullover

Shoulder Press with Squats

Wide and Narrow Grip Pull-ups

Bicep Curls with Both Arms and
    Elbows Away from Body

Tricep Dips

Supine Heel Drop

Abdominal Crunches on the Ball

Bicycle Maneuver

Supermans

Wondering what the next steps are? This could be the toughest stage of all because it means staying motivated. You want to be healthy for your whole life for all the reasons you already know: to ward off heart disease, diabetes, cancer, stroke, osteoporosis . . . the list goes on and on.

The most important step for you now is to set new goals or to reset your old ones. We discussed setting goals at great length in the Starting Out section of this book. But in case you need a refresher, a quick recap and some suggestions for setting new goals follow.

Make sure to make your goals SMART:

S = Specific

M = Measurable

A = Attainable

R = Realistic

T = Timed

Now that you are married—and looked and felt fabulous on your Big Day—ask yourself, "What do I want to tackle next?" Do you want to be able to run three miles without stopping? Run a 5K or a marathon? How about completing a walk for an organization that you feel passionate about? One event you may want to train for is the Danskin Triathlon, which is an amazing event for women. It is a mini-triathlon that allows all women to feel successful in a supportive, nurturing, caring environment. You can check it out online at www.danskin.com/danskinonline/triathlon.html. This incredible event has changed many women's lives, all in the name of charity; the proceeds go to the Breast Cancer Research Foundation.

But perhaps an organized race is too much. Instead, maybe your goal is to be able to play tag with your children or grandchildren, or to keep up with your husband on a mountain bike ride. Whatever the goal, keep moving toward it, and keep setting and resetting new goals that fit your life.

As you go forward with pursuing this new goal, be sure to get it in writing. Go ahead and write it down on this page:

My goal is to (do) _____ by (date) _____.
I will reach that goal by sticking to the following program I have designed for myself for the next six weeks. In six weeks I will evaluate my progress using regular fitness testing, make changes, and continue moving toward my end date.

Try to include all of the FITT principles you have learned: Frequency, Intensity, Time, and Type.

Use this space to write down your week-by-week goals:

WEEK	Mon	Tues	Wed	Thurs	Fri	Sat	Sun
25							
26							
27							
28							
29							
30							

Strength Training during Maintenance

Now that you've reached a desirable fitness level, here's a new level of strength training you can pursue. At 25 weeks, if you are ready for another challenge in your resistance program, try the routine outlined in this next section.

As stated earlier, you are welcome to use all the exercises in the three levels of the Healthy Bride program, keeping what you like and skipping what you do not. The important thing is to keep challenging your muscles for improvement. If you are happy with where you are, just mix things up enough to keep your body responding to the stimulus and make sure that your exercises are balanced. Work all major muscle groups, and work them together in the way they naturally are stressed in everyday life. This will keep your body in balance and help you avoid injury. All exercises included in this book are meant to reinforce daily life movements rather than isolate muscle groups individually.

As always, work on having perfect form. If your form breaks, you know that it's time to stop that particular exercise and move on to the next.

Whatever goal you choose, you have the tools you need to maintain a healthy fitness program. Having a workout buddy can help you stay on track. Recruit your bridesmaids, your mom, or you new hubby to work out with you, which will help you (and them) stay on your program long-term.

The key to sticking with your workout program is to make it enjoyable, set goals that are realistic, and commit to making exercise a part of your daily life. Remember, you made the commitment . . . for as long as you and your body both shall live.

Full Squats
(Works Legs and Glutes)

1. Stand with your legs shoulder width apart.

2. Shift all your body weight onto your heels.

3. Stick out your buttocks behind you as you lower your body toward the floor by bending your knees.

4. Continue to lower your body until your thighs are parallel to the floor.

5. Make sure you can see your toes past your knees at the lowest point in the exercise.

6. Return to standing position.

7. Repeat sequence.

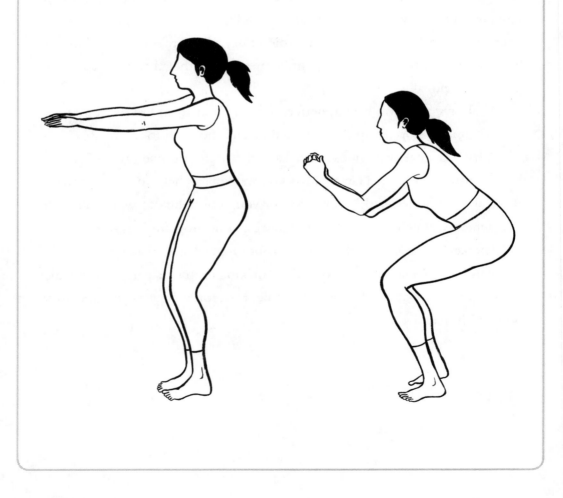

Walking Lunges with Dumbbells
(Works Hamstrings, Quadraceps, and Glutes)

USE THE SAME EXERCISE performed in Level Two (page 86), but now hold dumbbells in each hand as you step forward.

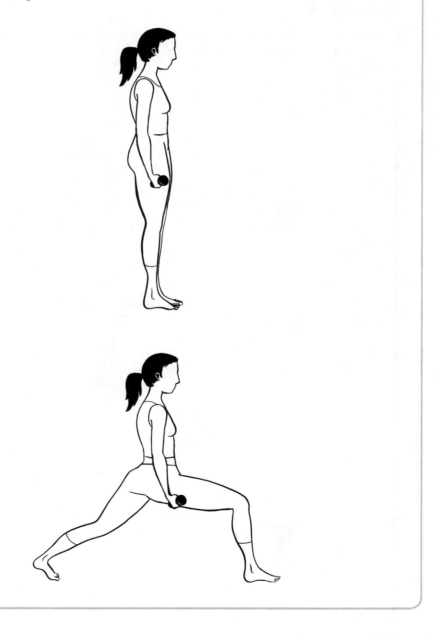

Hamstring Curls with Ball
(Works Hamstrings and Glutes)

1. Lie with your back on the floor with your feet on top of the ball. Your heels should be touching the center of the ball.

2. Extend your arms to the side of your body for support. Your arms should remain flat against the floor.

3. Lift your hips up so that your body is straight from your feet to your shoulders.

4. Hold this position until your feet remain steady on the ball.

5. Bring your feet toward your hips, rolling the ball toward you, keeping your hips up.

6. Return slowly to the starting position, and then repeat.

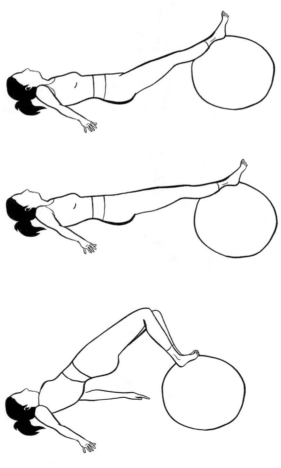

Jackknife on Ball
(Works the Lower Core)

1. From a standing position behind the ball, crouch down, place your abdomen on top of the ball, and roll forward until your hands reach the ground.

2. Walk out with your hands until your feet are flat on top of the ball and your body is in a firm straight line from head to toe.

3. Take a moment to steady your balance.

4. Roll your feet and knees toward your chest. Move slowly and in control.

5. Extend your legs back out to your starting position.

6. Repeat.

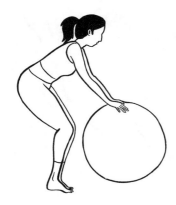
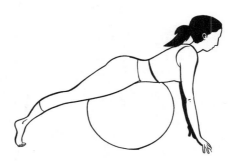

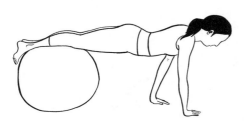
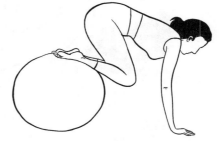

Adductor Ball Squeeze
(Works Inner Thighs, or Adductors)

USE THE SAME EXERCISE performed in Level Two (see page 89).

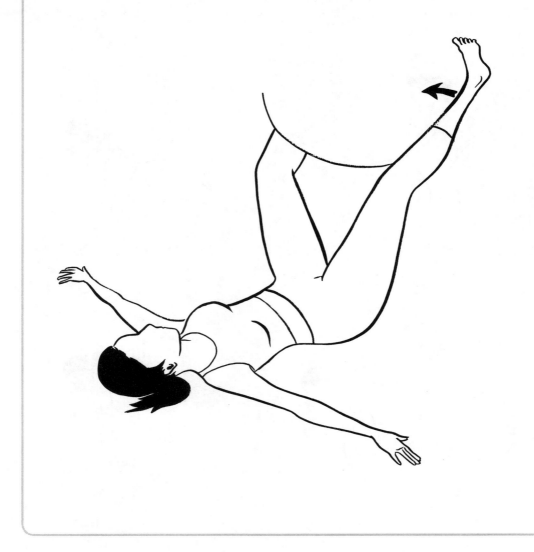

Side Leg Lifts with Band
(Works Outer Thighs, or Abductors)

USE THE SAME EXERCISE performed in Level Two (see page 88).

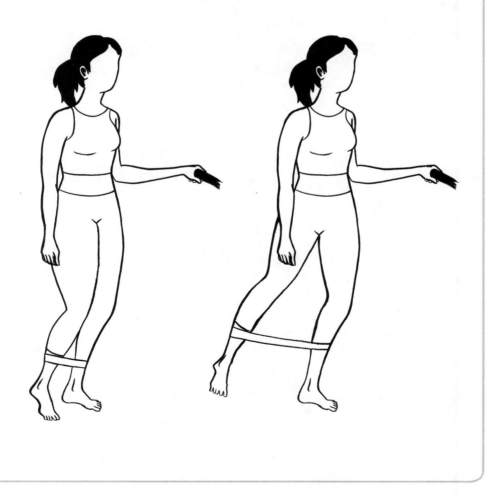

Lying Dumbbell Fly and Pullover
(Works Upper Body and Core)

1. Lie with the back of your head and your upper back supported by the ball.

2. Lift your hips up so that your body makes a straight line from your shoulders to your knees (in a bridging fashion).

3. Hold the dumbbells above your chest with your palms facing forward. This is your starting position.

4. Lower the dumbbells to either side. In an arced pattern, stop when your elbows are parallel to the floor.

5. Return to the start position.

6. Slowly lower the dumbbells over your head, with arms parallel to each other until your elbows are at ear level.

7. Your movements should be slow and controlled at all times.

8. Return to start position.

9. Repeat.

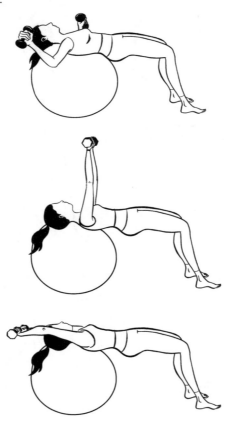

Shoulder Press with Squats
(Works Shoulders, Arms, and Legs)

FOR THIS EXERCISE, use dumbbells or substitute with a medicine ball or a bar if you wish.

1. Stand with your feet shoulder width apart, your knees slightly bent, and your toes forward.

2. Hold the weight or weights you're using at shoulder level. (If using a bar or dumbbells, your palms will face out.)

3. Press your arms over your head until they're extended but not locked.

4. While pressing up, squat with your lower body. (A half squat is fine, too, if you cannot comfortably squat all the way.)

5. Bring your arms back down.

6. Return to the upright position.

7. Repeat.

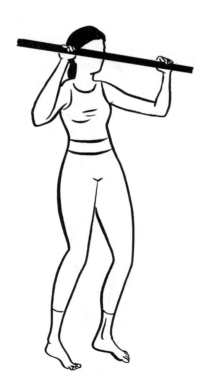
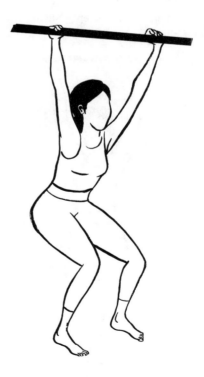

Wide and Narrow Grip Pull-ups
(Works Back Muscles)

YOUR GYM MAY HAVE an assisted pull-up machine. At home, you can use a chin-up bar. If you don't have a chin-up bar, go to a school or playground and use the jungle gym.

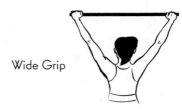

Wide Grip

1. Grip the bar with your arms slightly wider than elbow width for a wide pull, or at shoulder width for a narrow pull. The wide grip will be more difficult.

2. Make sure your palms face away from you.

3. Do not fully stretch your arms at the beginning; instead, keep a slight flex in your elbows.

4. Bring your chin above the bar within a one- to two-second count.

5. Slowly bring your body back down.

6. Use a spotter or put your feet on a chair, table, or ladder to assist your upward movement, but allow yourself to bring your own weight down with slow movements.

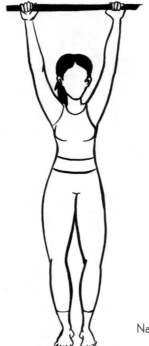

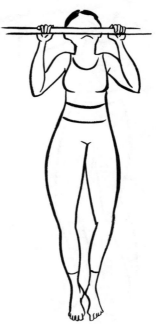

Narrow Grip Pull-up

Bicep Curls with Both Arms and Elbows Away from Body
(Works Biceps)

THIS IS THE SAME EXERCISE as the Bicep Curls in Level Two (see page 94). However, you must keep your elbows at about a 40-degree angle from your torso.

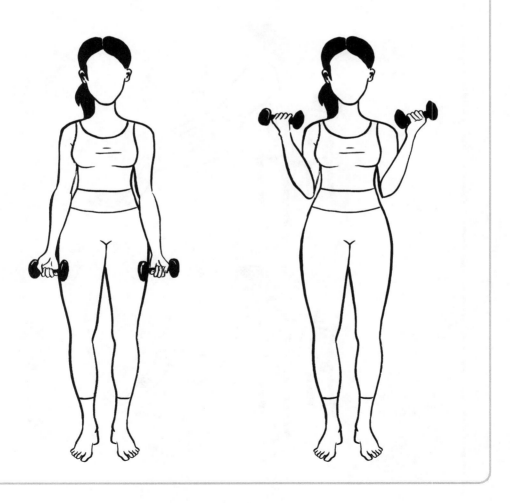

Tricep Dips
(Works Triceps)

1. Sit on the edge of a bench, step, or sturdy chair.

2. Position your hands beside your body on the edge of the bench (or whatever you're sitting on), fingers facing forward.

3. Lift your buttocks off the bench and lower them toward the floor by bending your arms at the elbows.

4. Make sure you stay perpendicular to the ground, and keep your back straight.

5. Don't push your hips forward.

6. Lift yourself back up by straightening your arms. Be sure to keep your arms close to your body throughout the exercise.

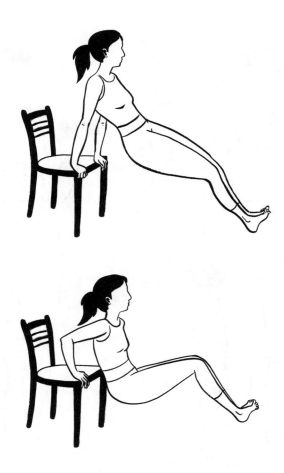

Supine Heel Drop
(Works Inner Abdominal Muscles)

USE THE SAME EXERCISE you did in Level Two (see page 96).

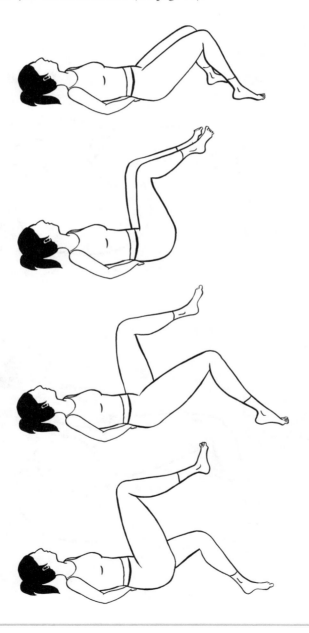

Abdominal Crunches on Ball
(Works Abs and Neck)

USE THE SAME EXERCISE you used in Levels One and Two (see page 67).

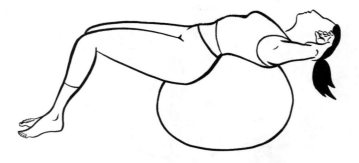

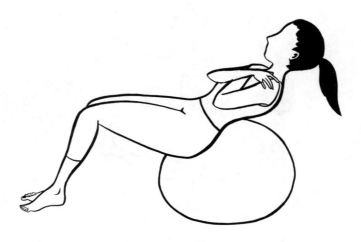

Bicycle Maneuver
(Works Abdominal Oblique Muscles)

USE THE SAME EXERCISE you did in Level One (see page 68).

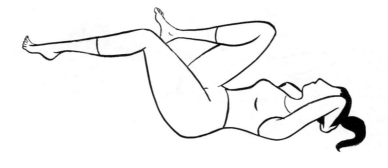

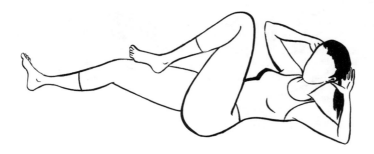

Supermans
(Works Back)

1. Lie on the floor with arms over your head and your legs straight.

2. Lift all four limbs as high off the floor as possible at the same time.

3. Hold to the count of three.

4. Relax.

5. Repeat.

6. Do 10 and work up to two sets.

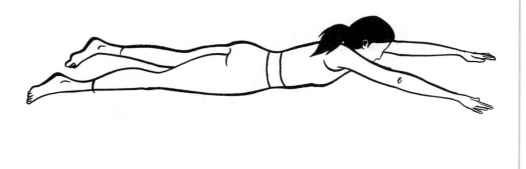

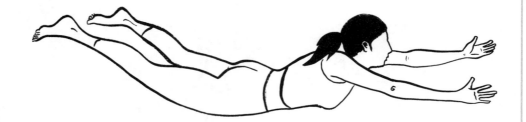

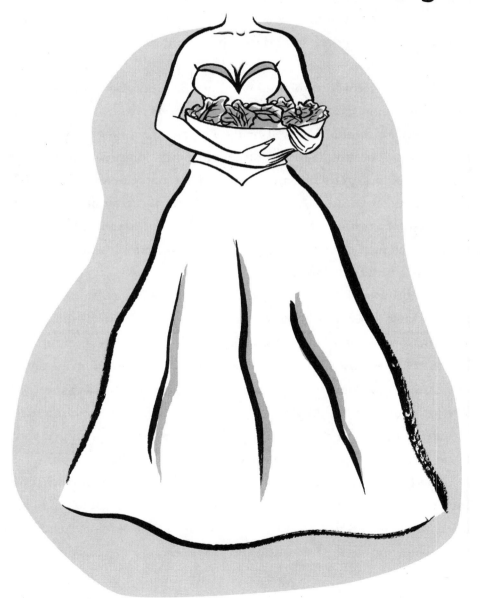

Part Three
The Healthy Bride
Nutrition Program

Marriage is a time of change and anticipation.

This part of the book describes the dietary changes that will lead you on the path to better health and, as a result, additional happiness.

Nutrition is usually associated with specific foods and calories. However, healthy nutrition is a lifestyle choice that supports your overall emotional health, physical health, and well-being. This part of the book will focus on maintaining a healthy diet as a bride and wife, along with all the factors that contribute to good nutrition. Included are strategies for making lifelong dietary changes. Ideal body weight is one factor in determining nutritional goals. Setting a realistic weight is important for your health and mental well-being. We all have distinct eating personalities to confront and manage when developing better nutritional habits.

As a bride-to-be, you may be feeling vulnerable and looking for fast results. Don't expect this book to provide any miracle cures or quick fixes to your diet or weight. Many popular diet books claim you can improve your health or lose weight if you follow their specific diet. However, one diet does not fit all. In this nutrition program, we will provide you with the tools to develop your own healthy dietary habits that will work for your lifestyle for months and years to come. This is a positive, long-term program that you can bring to your marriage as you develop and combine your meal plans.

The purpose of these nutritional chapters is not to tell you what to eat each day but to teach you how to eat better and make healthy food choices based on your personal food preferences. Once you develop dietary habits that include quality food selection and proper eating patterns, you're on your way to attaining an optimal weight to support your lifestyle, while lowering your risk of chronic disease.

To get the most from this part of the book, read through it once, and then go back to the "Create Meal Plans" chapter to practice what you have learned.

Before You Begin This Program

If you have any specific health issues, such as high blood pressure, high cholesterol, diabetes, or food allergies, the information given in this part of the book will still be beneficial, but you also should see a nutritionist to help you address your specific needs. In fact, all of us should see a nutritionist at least once in our lives to have our diets assessed and to ensure we have no potential health issues stemming from nutritional deficiencies.

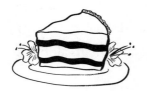

CHAPTER 11

Assess Your Nutritional Needs

As a bride, your motivation for making positive changes in your life is high at this time. Whether your wedding is next week or one year away, don't procrastinate. Seize the moment! Start making dietary changes now. You've taken the first step by getting this book, which means you have a plan in mind and instructions in hand.

In trying to look your best for your wedding day, it is tempting to go for quick fixes or crash diets. Don't fall for the trendy diets. Instead, seek long-term change; your body will thank you. Marriage is a commitment for the long term. Why not make the same commitment to healthy nutrition habits? This is not a time to make dramatic changes that may affect your health. Making small changes and adjustments along the way is the best approach for developing new habits.

One bride told me she almost passed out on her wedding day from the extremely low-calorie diet she put herself on to be skinny for her Big Day. I've seen too many brides desperate for this type of fast weight loss; don't fall into this trap. Going on such a poor nutritional "diet" is not a good idea, especially given the high stress of the wedding and the significance of the day. Wouldn't you want to be fully conscious and feeling your best throughout the ceremony and celebration? Your fiancé and family already love you for who you are.

Be reasonable about what you can accomplish and be comfortable with for your wedding day. Crash dieting or extremely low-calorie diets are not worth the health consequences. Besides, with crash diets the weight often returns in even less time than you were on the diet and may surpass the number of pounds you lost.

Be patient with yourself; dietary changes take time. Think about how long it took you to develop your current eating habits. Your ultimate goal is to implement a plan that will take you through the rest of your life. Also, keep in mind that this is the time to develop good nutrition habits you can later pass on to your new husband, your family, his family, and even your children (if you choose to have them). The idea is to learn to enjoy and appreciate foods that are healthy for you and your family.

When planning their wedding, most brides begin six months to one year before the Big Day. Besides planning for your wedding, why not plan for better nutritional habits, too? One year before the wedding is an ideal time to begin making dietary changes, whether it's for weight loss or just to improve your health and energy. Making minor changes in what you eat is easier than completely overhauling your diet. Allow for small changes as you develop new tastes and habits in your grocery shopping and food preparation. You have a time frame and specific deadlines for wedding planning; develop the same plan for dietary changes.

Keep in mind that you are also making some big lifestyle changes, too— for one thing, intertwining your life with that of the man you love. Set reasonable and attainable goals for your dietary changes. This is a good time to get support from your fiancé, family, and friends. They already will be involved in your wedding, so why not have them join you in your dietary progress? By doing so, you just may have the best-looking and most healthy wedding party. Successful programs for sustaining change are made when family and friends are involved in a positive way.

Don't let these changes slip after the wedding. Just as you will have to continue to work on your relationship, continue to improve your dietary habits. Remember, good nutrition is a lifelong commitment, too.

Your Healthy Body Weight

Ideal body weight does not mean fitting into a specific wedding-dress size. Determining an ideal body weight for your body type can be difficult. We are all unique in our bone structure and genetics, so you may not be able to fit into a size 6 pair of pants without jeopardizing your health or setting yourself up for failure. Plus, no standard for clothing sizes exists, so you may fit into a size 10 with one designer and a size 8 with another.

Instead of trying to make your body fit the dress, find a wedding dress that accentuates your unique shape and is comfortable. Your body will move toward a healthy, natural shape with this nutrition program. We don't all have the same bone structure as a supermodel or mannequin. Our lean body mass—the weight of our bones, organs, and muscles—may cause us to weigh more and still be healthy and fit. In other words, we don't always fit into a specific weight category found on standard health charts.

The best strategy for attaining your ideal weight is to have good nutrition, control your portion sizes, and exercise. This will allow your body to find its natural and healthy weight. It's a difficult approach to take with all the media focus on ultra-thin models and movie stars. Looking through bridal magazines or watching TV, especially reality shows, gives us a skewed perspective of the ideal body weight or natural shape. A healthy body weight is a weight at which you feel your best as you go about your daily life, not a weight that matches an ideal imposed on you by the media. What you want to focus on is finding a realistic weight that promotes optimal health and well-being. When you feel good, you will look good, too.

Because we all have different body types with varying percentages of lean and fat mass, the more accurate determination of health is to measure your body composition. Body composition measured by skin-fold calipers or hydrostatic weighing to determine your percentage of body fat is a better determination of health than the actual weight your bathroom scale reads.

(Skin-fold calipers assess body fat by measuring the thickness of skin folds at standardized sites on the body. Hydrostatic weighing, also known as underwater weighing, assesses body fat by the relationship between normal body weight and underwater weight.) The combination of good nutrition and exercise naturally leads to a healthy body composition. Most health clubs and some physicians can perform body composition measurements to determine a healthy lean mass for your particular body. This is a better determination of long-term health and one that can lower your risk of chronic disease.

When altering your diet, always ask yourself these key questions: How do I feel? Do I have enough energy? Am I prone to illness?

In my practice, I've seen brides who manage to reach what they consider an ideal body weight but couldn't maintain it because they felt weak and unhealthy. This is your body telling you this is not a good weight for you. You may *look* great according to some external ideal, but you may *feel* awful. The following chapters will guide you through the process of improving your nutrition and attaining your healthy body weight to feel your best.

Identify Your Eating Personality

Your eating personality can be a roadblock to healthy nutrition. In addition, your eating personality may dominate your eating habits during times of high stress. Pay close attention to this as you approach your wedding day. What is your eating personality? Following are a few examples of eating personalities that usually lead to overconsumption of calories. Do any of these sound like you?

- **Stress eater:** "When I'm really stressed out, eating helps me conquer that stress."

- **Boredom eater:** "When there's nothing to do and I'm bored, eating helps fill the void."

- **Reward eater:** "I've had such a rough day [or week or year], I deserve to eat this."

- **Depressed eater:** "When I'm down, I feel better by eating."

- **Social eater:** "When I'm at social gatherings, there's so much food around and so much going on, I find myself eating constantly without even noticing it."

No matter what your eating personality, always ask yourself what your motivations for eating may be. All the eating personalities just mentioned are emotionally based, which can lead to unhealthy eating habits or possibly eating disorders.

Also, ask yourself if it's been a while since you've last eaten. In some instances of high stress, you may just need to eat. Ever find yourself snapping at friends or family members if you've skipped a meal? Low blood sugar from lack of food can cause symptoms of depression, anxiety, and stress. Recognize if your behavior is negatively affected by low blood sugar, and if so, have a healthy snack or meal to curb it.

No doubt eating is an emotionally satisfying experience, but consider your real motivations for eating. It is key that you learn the difference between eating for an emotional need and eating for a physical need. Understanding your eating personality is the first step toward positive change.

Check in with yourself and gauge your emotional state when you are eating. This is how you can be more aware of what is really going on with yourself. Deal with your emotional state and find alternatives to food that satisfy your eating personality. Learn to make yourself a priority. Treat yourself to a soothing cup of herbal tea, a massage, or a hot bath. Be creative; find a no-calorie alternative to placate your eating personality. Find strategies to decompress, and accept that planning your wedding will be a stressful time of dealing with your own expectations and those of family. If stress levels are outrageously high or if you have or think you may have an eating disorder, you may want to seek a counselor for professional support.

Learn to Confront Cravings and Deprivation

OK, let's fast-forward a few weeks. Say you've been doing well on your new nutrition program. But you've really been missing something you used to eat more of, perhaps your favorite chocolate-chip cookie or potato chips. If you've been doing well and you think you're going to fall off the wagon and go hog wild, you'd better give in to this craving early on before it takes over. In my experience, it's better to have a little bit of something to satisfy your craving than to let the craving grow until you can't control how much you eat. It's OK to give in to a craving every so often as long as you don't overdo it.

If you think depriving yourself of a certain food or eating a specific food is going to trigger a total binge, you may need to consult a professional counselor or therapist. This is nothing to be ashamed of, especially because you may be unknowingly dealing with more issues than just self-control.

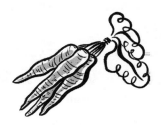

CHAPTER 12

How to Eat Properly

Eating patterns are defined by how often and when you eat. This is as important as what you eat. In your busy life of meeting the daily demands of wedding preparations, appointments, traveling, and obligations, it's easy to forget to eat or to be caught off guard by hunger.

Ever notice how moms are so great about packing snacks for children to ensure that they eat regularly, don't get grouchy, and don't become out of control? If busy moms can do this for their kids, you should be able to do this for yourself. You need to feed yourself regularly to maintain a constant level of nutrients and energy. Doing so will also help regulate your mood. And you'll need a lot of mood support to survive wedding preparations.

Some of us need to eat more often, depending on our metabolism and the type of meal or snack that we had. Add eating times for meals and snacks to the same schedule you use for the photographer, caterer, or any other appointment during your day. Incorporating your food schedule into your daily plans will keep hunger under control.

Waiting too long to eat can set you up for craving unhealthy foods and can reduce your ability to make wise food choices. How often you eat can make the difference in how many calories you will consume in a day. This strategy is called "*eating to lose weight.*" Needing a quick fix causes a desperation that makes for poor nutrition choices and sets the stage for overeating. Instead, avoid skipping breakfast, and try to have some protein with each of your meals and snacks to preempt unhealthy cravings.

Plan ahead and beware of situations where you won't have reasonable food choices. Eating at appropriate intervals of three to four hours prevents overeating and making unwise food choices. Don't wait until extreme hunger hits. Don't let yourself become that screaming, out-of-control child; instead, be prepared and become that composed bride-to-be.

How many times have you had a meal and couldn't remember much about it? Although this is not ideal, it's easy enough to remedy. The way you eat is important; you should eat slowly and chew your food well. This gives your body a chance to realize it is full. It can take up to 20 minutes for your body to register that it's had enough. Chewing food thoroughly assists in digestion and allows you to absorb more nutrients from the food. Think of this as the "Zen" of eating. Become more self-aware while eating. This will allow you and your body to savor the meal and appreciate its full nutritional value.

The following are some basic strategies for acquiring good eating patterns:

- Plan a variety of meals and snacks in advance and set a schedule to eat every three to four hours to keep hunger attacks and low energy at bay.

- Prepare a list before grocery shopping and stick to it. This will help you be a more efficient shopper, prevent impulse buys, and keep a well-stocked kitchen.

- Prepare food shortly after your shopping trip. Wash, cut, and chop vegetables for salads, stir-fries, or snacks. Store prepped foods in airtight containers until they're ready to use. Having foods prepped and readily available for snacks and meal preparation prevents the urge to eat unhealthy snacks and fast foods.

- Pack food for work, a long drive, school, or wherever you'll be. Buy sealable snack baggies or small containers for easy grab-and-go foods.

- Use the balanced food pyramid and suggested serving sizes in Appendix A to determine your dietary needs and food choices.

- Measure all foods to get a better idea of how much food you are eating. People have a common tendency to underestimate serving sizes. You'd be surprised at how portion sizes can grow with "guesstimation." After a while, you'll be able to gauge your portion sizes more accurately without measuring them.

Eating Survival Skills for Social Gatherings

As a bride-to-be, expect and plan ahead for the inevitable gatherings you'll attend, such as engagement parties, bridal showers, and other celebrations. These gatherings can be fraught with so many distractions, from people you haven't seen in a while to endless photo opportunities, that you usually don't get to eat a balanced meal. Don't get so caught up with the socializing, eating, and drinking that you lose track of how much food or drink you've had. Bring more awareness to your food and beverage intake. At the same time, don't let a new nutrition plan spoil your fun. This section will help you navigate these events with strategies for making wise food choices and lowering your calorie intake.

Here are a few tips for surviving the party-food situation:

- Never arrive at a party on an empty stomach. By doing so, you set yourself up for binging on high-calorie, high-fat foods. Instead, have a small, balanced snack before arriving. Besides, wouldn't you want the pictures to show you smiling and enjoying the company of friends and family rather than caught with a mouthful of food?

- Situate yourself away from the buffet table or food area. Staying close to the food can set you up for mindless snacking.

- Scope out the buffet selection before filling your plate. This way you can decide in advance what the healthier choices are and what to avoid.

- If you are close to the people throwing the party, let them know in advance about your health goals for your wedding and ask them to have healthy options available.

- Spend more time socializing. You'll have the opportunity to learn so much more about your friends and future family.

- Enjoy the special-occasion foods that normally would not be available to you. Watch portion sizes and savor the special occasion for what it is.

- No matter what you are eating, take your time with it. Chew well to aid digestion and really taste (and enjoy) what you're eating.

Dining Out: Tips to Guide You through the Menu

Because some of your pre-wedding gatherings may occur at restaurants, here are a few pointers for selecting and ordering healthy meals while dining out.

High-fat foods are higher in calories, and a high-fat diet can lead to increased risk of chronic disease. With that in mind, use the following examples for reducing fat when dining out. To lower your fat intake:

- Avoid cream- or cheese-based sauces or soups. Order broth- or tomato-based sauces or soups instead.

- Limit or avoid eating chips and bread with butter before the meal.

- Choose fish and poultry over red meats, as the latter are higher in saturated fat.

- Trim off visible fat from meat and remove skin from poultry before eating.

- Reduce, replace, or avoid high-fat condiments or additions such as sour cream, cheese, bacon, and butter. For example, have a sandwich with mustard instead of mayonnaise, or just have a small amount of mayonnaise on it.

- Avoid deep-fried foods such as french fries, fried noodles, and breaded items. Look for grilled, baked, roasted, broiled, steamed, poached, or sautéed items.

- Ask for salad dressing on the side so that you can control the amount of dressing on your salad.

• Request that foods be prepared with less oil or butter.

To reduce your calorie intake:

• Try ordering an appetizer and salad instead of a main course.

• Share your entrée with your dining companions.

• Don't be afraid to ask questions or ask for healthier substitutions. Be assertive when ordering; it lets the restaurant know that you care about your health, and it may prompt them to put healthier options on the menu.

• Stop eating once you are full and request a take-home container for the rest.

• When your dish arrives, visualize immediately how much you plan to eat and how much you plan to take home. You can even ask for a take-home container in advance and fill it before eating.

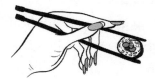

CHAPTER 13

Develop Nutrition Know-how

Your relationship with food is an ongoing work in progress, just as your relationship with your husband-to-be is. Some days are better than others, and you soldier on regardless of setbacks and continue to improve the relationship. As you gather more insight, your confidence and ability to find a comfortable balance in your newly merged lives become more natural. The same is true for your relationship with food and your knowledge of good nutrition.

We commonly focus on calories when thinking about diet; a "diet" is not the best term to use because it gives the impression of eating a certain way until you reach a desired weight. For the stereotypical diet, in which daily menus are strictly regimented, you will not and are not capable of maintaining weight loss for the long term. An extreme example is the "grapefruit diet," in which you eat only grapefruit. This is a very limited diet and is not nutritionally sound. You may lose a little or even a lot of weight on this diet, but at some point you will return to your old routine, and the weight will come back.

So-called "diets" should not be temporary if you want to maintain a healthy weight. A better strategy is to aim for healthy nutrition as a long-term commitment. Weight cycling—repeatedly gaining and losing weight—can be stressful on the body and hard on the pocketbook—in terms of food and clothing. Do consider your calorie intake. It is most important to ensure that you eat the right balance of protein, carbohydrates, fat (yes, we do need fat), vitamins, and minerals. Many times when we cut calories, we cut vital nutrients. With those considerations in mind, here are some terms and concepts that will help you develop your nutrition know-how and ensure you get the right balance of nutrients.

Energy Balance

Proper weight maintenance is related to the balance of calories eaten to calories burned. *Energy balance* occurs when the calories eaten and the calories burned are equal. To maintain your weight, energy balance is absolutely necessary. Eating too many calories and burning too little will lead to weight gain. Creating a calorie deficit is the key to weight loss.

By following the Healthy Bride workout and nutrition programs, you will be burning more calories and eating fewer calories. The proportions of protein, carbohydrate, and fat you eat do not determine energy balance. However, if you consume more calories than you can burn, you won't have a calorie deficit—and you won't lose weight. Tricking yourself into consuming fewer calories with a balanced combination of eating nutrient-dense foods (defined in the following pages) and feeling satiated for longer is the secret to weight loss.

Calorie-dense vs. Nutrient-dense Foods

Calorie-dense foods tend to pack a lot of calories with little nutrition. They are usually highly refined, meaning that many of the nutrients and fiber are removed or missing. Examples of calorie-dense foods are candy, white bread, donuts, scones, cookies, and cakes. Alternatively, *nutrient-dense* foods are less refined and contain more nutrients and fiber, which makes for fewer calories. Examples of nutrient-dense foods are whole-wheat bread (or any whole-grain food), fruits, and vegetables. When you consume more nutrient-dense foods, you consume fewer calories and increase your nutrient and fiber intake.

So, focus instead on nutrient-dense foods. When our nutritional needs are being met, we tend to feel better and eat better. A baked scone is an example of a calorie-dense food; it can add up to 500+ calories and offers little nutritional value. On the other hand, a lower-calorie, higher-nutrient alternative such as a bowl of whole-grain cereal with milk and fresh fruit could have half the calories. The baked scone consists mainly of refined carbohydrates (in the form of white flour), sugar, and fat; however, the bowl of cereal with fruit and milk contains protein, high amounts of fiber, vitamins, minerals, and phytonutrients. (Phytonutrients are plant nutrients that come from fruits, vegetables, and whole grains and promote good health.) Recognize and choose nutrient-dense foods more often to lower your calorie intake.

Whole Foods vs. Processed Foods

Whole foods are naturally nutrient-dense and contain a lower amount of calories. These foods closely resemble the way they occur in nature—in other words, they have not been processed. Fresh fruits, vegetables, and whole grains are examples of "whole foods" that retain their original nutrients.

Processed foods, on the other hand, have been manipulated in ways that usually take away the natural nutrients and turn the foods into something far removed from the way nature created them. A prime example of a processed food is refined wheat flour, also known as white flour, in which the bran and germ have been removed, leaving a product that has less fiber and nutrients. Other processed foods include fast foods and packaged foods. Fast foods and packaged foods are usually highly processed with chemical additives and preservatives that are not healthy.

The benefits of whole foods are endless: They satiate you for longer periods of time, they have exceptional nutritional value, and they provide fewer calories than processed foods. For balanced meals and snacks, eat whole foods–based meals and snacks that consist of carbohydrates, protein, and a little fat. You will notice a difference in your health and energy level without feeling deprived of the processed or refined foods you once craved.

Quick-fix and Low-carb Diets

Television ads and magazines offer a multitude of quick-fix solutions for weight loss, from low-carb diets to grapefruit diets to miracle supplements in the forms of drinks, pills, powders, and herbs. With your wedding coming up, such quick weight-loss solutions will certainly be tempting. But these quick fixes often have few or no health advantages, may be ineffective, and can be dangerous if not used properly.

You should not try to follow any diet that focuses too much on one food group while eliminating others. Save money for your future; don't spend it on any nutritional supplement that claims to help you lose weight. There is no such thing as a weight-loss pill. In fact, to date, there is no scientific evidence that supports any type of weight-loss supplement, no matter what all those ads say. Don't sacrifice your health (not to mention your time and money) for any quick fix for weight loss. You have too much to look forward to.

With all the attention on carbohydrates, more needs to be said about the Atkins Diet, the South Beach Diet, and all other low-carb alternatives. You'd have to be living in a cave or on a deserted island to not get caught up in the hoopla of low-carb diets. The main reason people lose weight on low-carb diets is they decrease or limit their intake of refined carbohydrates. These refined carbohydrates are the sugars and refined flours in white bread, pastries, and cookies. As mentioned earlier in this chapter, because these are all high-calorie foods, taking them away also means taking away their high calories, which will contribute to weight loss. So, that part of these low-carb plans is actually quite beneficial.

However, most low-carb diets are also high in fat and protein. Another reason to avoid these diets is that they usually focus on eating animal protein, which leads to a high intake of saturated fat. High intake of saturated fats may raise your cholesterol and triglyceride levels, which in turn leads to increased risk of chronic disease. Protein in excess can also turn into fat because it contains high amounts of calories, too.

Instead, gain the benefits of the low-carb hype by cutting refined carbohydrates and eating lean protein from animal and/or vegetable sources while reducing fat. This combination improves satiety, which will keep you from overeating or snacking too often.

It's not a good idea to stay on these low-carb diets too long, and you should never completely eliminate all carbs from your diet. You may end up with some nutritional deficiencies because unrefined carbohydrates ("good carbohydrates") contain vital nutrients that cannot be found in other foods; these carbs are a primary fuel source for your body . . . especially the muscles. Most people on these diets cannot sustain the low-carb, high-protein eating regimen for very long. Many have reported feeling weak and lethargic, and many have said they've experienced mood swings and/or digestive issues. Low-carb diets are not a good option for the long term.

Also, I cannot state this more strongly: *Eating the right carbohydrates is not bad for you and will not make you fat.* The right carbohydrates are actually good for you, as you will learn in the next chapter. In fact, if you limit some types of carbohydrates, you may end up with nutritional deficiencies and/or digestive issues such as constipation from lack of fiber. Research continues to support a balanced diet for maintaining long-term weight loss. A low-carb diet will only be a temporary quick fix and is not worth the health risks.

One more caution about quick-fix diets: Ever notice how low-carb, high-protein diets recommend taking special supplements while you're on the diet? Besides trying to get you to buy more specialty products, they are trying to fill the gaps of missing nutrients from a limited diet, further proving that low-carb diets are often unbalanced. (To see for yourself, check out the balanced food pyramid provided in Appendix A to see how much you'd be missing in a low-carb diet.)

Multivitamins

Finally, don't rely on multivitamins to make up for poor eating. Multivitamins vary greatly in terms of quality, as does your ability to absorb the nutrients from the supplements themselves. Many valuable phytonutrients are not included in multivitamins. Through natural unprocessed food, Mother Nature has a way of presenting the right quantity and balance of nutrients for optimal absorption, another reason why whole foods are so nutritionally valuable. All this said, multivitamins can provide some necessary nutrients, but use them only as a supplement and not as a substitute for eating well.

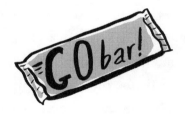

CHAPTER 14

Anatomy of a Healthy Diet

To understand what healthy nutrition is, you need to understand the components of various foods and the benefits that they provide. First of all, there is no single completely balanced food. The food industry would like you to think you can live on nutrition bars, protein-powder drinks, and fortified cereals. Don't believe it. You will do better to eat a variety of foods in the right proportions to get the most nutritional value. Use this section along with the balanced food pyramid and average serving sizes in Appendix A as guides to making your food selections. Branch out and seek new healthy foods that you might not otherwise try. And remember, variety is the spice of life *and* nutrition, so try not to eat the same thing day after day. Besides being boring and limiting in nutrients, a lack of variety means you're missing a whole world of foods and flavors to try.

The following sections define the components of the various foods that comprise a healthy diet. Use this information to help you choose foods that will provide the most diversity of nutrients that make up a balanced diet.

Fuel Up on Carbohydrates

Carbohydrates are the sugars, starches, and fiber found in fruits, vegetables, grains, and dairy products. We need carbohydrates for energy. Carbohydrates break down to form glucose (also called "blood sugar"), which provides energy for your muscles, brain, and other tissues. This is your primary fuel, and it's especially important for supporting you throughout your workout program as well as through your wedding preparations and wedding day. Ever try to think straight or make difficult decisions on an empty stomach? Then you know it's no easy task. That's your brain telling you it's low in glucose, and therefore, low in carbohydrates.

A healthy bride needs to select the right carbohydrates to sustain energy and support weight loss. Simple, refined carbohydrates such as refined sugar and refined flours tend to be white—you know, the bad stuff in all those cookies, pies, and pastries we love. Eating too much of these will make you gain weight. They also have little nutritional value and provide little satiety over the long run.

On the other hand, breads, rice, pasta, crackers, and cereals are traditionally classified as complex carbohydrates. Know that complex carbohydrates can be made of refined grains. A better distinction to make is whether the complex carbohydrate is made from whole or refined grains. In other words, is it a whole food or a processed food?

Refined Carbohydrates to Avoid or Limit

The following is a list of simple/refined carbohydrates that have lower nutritional value and can contribute to weight gain.

- White bread
- White rice
- White rolls
- Pasta made with semolina or wheat flour (both refined grains)
- Cookie
- Pastries
- White sugar
- Brown sugar
- Refined grain crackers such as saltines
- High-fructose corn syrup and other refined sweeteners

These foods are highly processed with little or no fiber and few nutrients. They are calorie-dense, will digest quickly and easily, and will create a spike and then drop in blood-glucose levels. This wreaks havoc on your energy and/or emotions, putting you on a roller coaster of highs and lows—from feeling energetic, happy, or anxious to feeling extremely fatigued or depressed. Refined carbohydrates are notorious for providing a quick fix to hunger that doesn't last long and leaves you wanting to eat more.

In addition, it is easy to overeat refined carbohydrates and gain weight from the concentrated calories. Ever notice how you can eat almost a whole loaf of freshly baked white bread? You'd be hard-pressed to do the same with a whole-grain loaf. Refined grains are not good for maintaining satiety, which is why we often eat too much and gain weight with these.

Healthy Unrefined Carbohydrates

The following are whole-grain carbohydrates that are high in fiber and nutrients that will make you feel full longer.

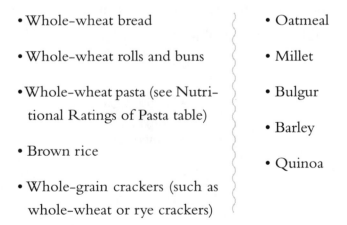

- Whole-wheat bread

- Whole-wheat rolls and buns

- Whole-wheat pasta (see Nutritional Ratings of Pasta table)

- Brown rice

- Whole-grain crackers (such as whole-wheat or rye crackers)

- Oatmeal

- Millet

- Bulgur

- Barley

- Quinoa

All the foods just listed are whole foods. The unrefined/whole grain carbohydrates pack in a lot more nutrition than their refined counterparts. They will digest slowly, lead to a gradual release of glucose, and will sustain you for

Nutritional Ratings of Pasta

Nutritional Rating	Type of Pasta/Noodles	Comments
LOW	Durum wheat, semolina, rice, and vegetable	These are all refined grain products that are of low nutritional value. The processing of the grains leaves the product low in fiber and nutrients. Vegetable pastas such as spinach and tomato are usually made with refined wheat. The colors of these pastas come from vegetable powder, which does little to increase the nutritional value.
MEDIUM	Multigrain, blended, and low-carb	The major ingredient in these products is usually refined wheat with the addition of a variety of legume flours, flaxseed, wheat germs and/or wheat bran. These additions increase the fiber and nutrients. Since the main ingredient is refined wheat, nutrients and fiber will be lower than a whole-grain product. Some low-carb pastas will have little or no wheat flour and mainly consist of legume flour (soy, lentil, and/or garbanzo); these are higher in protein. Don't expect these low-carb pastas to taste like conventional pastas. The pastas listed here are better choices than completely refined grain pastas.
HIGH	Whole wheat, whole durum wheat, brown rice, corn, quinoa, spelt, and kamut	These are all whole grains. The minimal processing of these grains preserves the naturally occurring nutrients and fiber. These are the best choices for pasta.

longer. Set a goal of eating 6–11 servings per day of whole-grain foods. (See Appendix A for serving sizes.) Eat a variety of these foods to get a wide array of nutrients in your diet. Stick with high-quality whole grains and avoid the refined grains.

If you're feeling adventurous and want to expand your repertoire of grains, quinoa (pronounced "keen-wa"), millet, and amaranth can be made into a nice hot cereal. (See the recipes in Appendix B for ideas on how to prepare these grains.) These grains are high in protein and have plenty of nutrients and fiber.

Unfortunately, you do need to make a conscious effort to increase whole grains in your diet. Although restaurants and grocery stores traditionally haven't featured these items, more and more grocery stores are offering such items today.

For example, more whole-wheat pastas and brown-rice products are showing up on grocery-store shelves and in bulk-food aisles than in years past. In part this is because of the low-carb fad; check the labels of some low-carb pastas and you'll find that they tend to be made with whole-wheat flour. High-fiber foods tend to be lower in so-called net carbs because the fiber is not factored in. (FYI, no true definition of net carbs exists, so you can't go by what the packaging advertises.) Evidently, these whole grains tend to be lower in total carbohydrates because of their high-fiber and higher protein content.

A word of warning: Some low-carb products are not low-calorie and taste awful because of the bean flours added to boost the protein content. This "manipulation" takes the food farther from being either a real or whole food. So whenever you're grocery shopping, read the ingredients list and look for whole grains. Although it takes more time, it's worth the effort to become more familiar with the foods you are buying.

Suggested Vegetables

Here are a few of many healthy vegetables to incorporate into your diet:

- Leafy greens (bok choy and other Asian greens, kale, chard, and collards)

- Cabbage (purple/red, green, napa, and savoy)

- Broccoli

- Green- and red-leaf lettuce

- Romaine

- Spinach

- Sweet potatoes and yams

- Carrots

- Green beans

- Sweet bell peppers (red, green, yellow, and orange)

In addition to grain products, vegetables and fruits are in the carbohydrate category. They provide fiber and many phytonutrients (in the form of antioxidants). Choose from a wide selection of vegetables and try to buy seasonally for the most nutrition. Vegetables have virtually no fat and are very low in calories. Starchy vegetables such as peas, potatoes, corn, sweet potatoes, and yams tend to be higher in calories per serving than nonstarchy vegetables. It doesn't mean that they are bad for you; they are still nutritious but higher in calories. Keep starchy vegetables to less than two servings per day for weight loss. You can have an unlimited variety of nonstarchy vegetables per day because they are low in calories and high in nutrients.

Suggested Fruits

Here is a list of some healthy fruits to have in your Healthy Bride nutrition program.

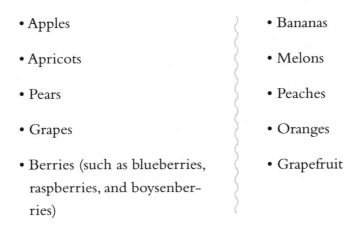

- Apples
- Apricots
- Pears
- Grapes
- Berries (such as blueberries, raspberries, and boysenberries)

- Bananas
- Melons
- Peaches
- Oranges
- Grapefruit

Fruits make excellent low-fat snack foods and sweet alternatives to refined-sugar products. Choose fruits in season because they will be fresher, more nutritious, and less expensive. Try to select from a variety of colors to increase your intake of various antioxidants. Eating whole fruit instead of drinking juice will provide you with additional fiber and fewer calories. Fruit juice usually has the fiber taken away, leaving only the concentrated juice, which is mostly sugar. An eight-ounce glass of orange juice can add up to 180 calories to your fruit intake, and it takes four or more oranges to make it. On the other hand, by eating one orange, you will ingest only 60 calories; plus, you will have more fiber and feel more satisfied (and therefore less hungry).

If you do drink juice, dilute it with water to lower the calories and increase your water intake. You will soon find that straight juice has become too sweet to your taste.

You may also want to begin drinking smoothies instead of juice. Smoothies are an excellent alternative when made with whole fruit. For a good starter in preparing your own smoothies, try the smoothie recipe in Appendix B.

Carbohydrate Plan

Carbohydrates should actually make up the majority of your calories; overall they should consist of 45–65 percent of your total food intake. If you exercise more than one hour per day, your carbohydrate needs will be in the higher range (closer to 65 percent). Have a small carbohydrate snack within 30 minutes of finishing your workout to replenish your muscle energy storage and to improve recovery. You'll notice the difference in your next workout session.

The recommended carbohydrates in this chapter are part of the main food groups of grains, fruits, and vegetables. When you incorporate these carbohydrate foods into your diet, you will get a great dose of essential nutrients and fiber. Essential nutrients are nutrients your body cannot make, so they must be taken in as food. Your body cannot survive without them. As an added bonus, you will be protecting yourself from chronic diseases such as cardiovascular disease, cancer, and diabetes. This will set you on the path to living happily and healthily ever after.

Dietary Fats

We've been trained to avoid fat, assuming that it is bad for us and will make us, in turn, fat. Dietary fat is actually quite necessary for maintaining good health. Your brain and nervous system cannot function without fat. The fats in food provide essential fats, or fats that the body cannot make and must be absorbed from our diet. We need dietary fat to digest and absorb fat-soluble vitamins, which support our vision, healthy skin, and bones. The fat-soluble vitamins are vitamins A, D, E, and K.

Per gram, fat has more calories (nine calories per gram) than protein or carbohydrates, which is why it's usually the first thing cut from a diet to lose weight. Historically, though, low-fat diets don't lead to weight loss. Low-fat diets were long thought to be the answer, but then we eliminated too much fat from our diets. As a culture, we got into trouble by replacing fat with too many carbohydrates. As a result, our health and waistlines suffered.

Many nonfat products replaced their fat content with refined carbohydrates, which compensated or overcompensated for the calories taken away by reducing the fat. (SnackWell's cookies were one of the first nonfat cookies on the market. Guess what? A lot of sugar was added to make them taste "good" without the fat.) These types of foods usually are not satisfying, and in the past, we mistakenly believed that we could not gain weight from them because they are low in fat or nonfat. The truth is they still contain calories that mainly come from sugar, and those calories can cause you to gain additional weight. Sometimes it's worth it to have a small amount of the real thing and really savor it, rather than overeating something that is a poor replacement. Have these foods in moderation and you will not feel deprived.

Many foods contain either good fats or bad fats, or both. This doesn't mean you can't have any of the bad fats and you should only eat the good fats—just keep the bad fats low in your diet. Besides, life would be really boring and bland without a balance between good and bad. But first, you need to know how to differentiate bad fats from good fats.

Bad Fats

Saturated fats are bad fats. Saturated fats have been implicated in heart disease (they can raise LDL cholesterol, or the "bad" cholesterol), cancer, and other diseases and ailments. Meats, full-fat cheese, and dairy products are high in saturated fats.

The other bad fats that have been getting lots of attention recently are *trans fats*, which are made from hydrogenated fats. You may see the terms "trans fat" and "hydrogenated fat" used interchangeably. Trans fats are chemically created by a process called *hydrogenation*, which makes a liquid vegetable oil into a solid fat that has a longer shelf life. It was originally thought that trans fat as in margarine would be a healthier replacement for the saturated fat in butter. As it turns out, it is not. Trans fats should be avoided completely because they are responsible for a much higher incidence of heart disease than saturated fats and have been known to raise LDL cholesterol (the "bad" cholesterol) and lower levels of HDL cholesterol (the "good" cholesterol).

These trans fats are found in shortening, baked goods, crackers, margarines, and deep-fried foods. Margarine made with trans fat is worse than the saturated fat in butter. If given a choice between margarine made with trans fat and butter, choose butter, using it in small amounts. In addition, we've always known that deep-fried foods are bad for us. Besides being high in calories, they are high in trans fat. Given this information, it is really best to avoid deep-fried foods altogether.

The good news is that many food manufacturers are starting to remove trans fat from their foods, so you will now see margarines with labels saying they are "trans fat–free" or they contain "no hydrogenated fats." Currently, the only way to determine whether your product contains trans fat is to look for "hydrogenated oils" or "hydrogenated shortening" in the ingredients list. More good news: As of 2006, trans fat is now required on the nutrition facts panel found on food labels. This is an invaluable tool for avoiding trans-fat intake.

Good Fats

Unsaturated fats such as polyunsaturated and monounsaturated fat are the good fats. Fish oils, olive oils, and avocado are high in unsaturated fats, and they are the naturally occurring fats in vegetables, nuts, and seeds.

The essential fats found in these foods are necessary for our bodies to function properly and to prevent chronic disease. Unsaturated fats provide the most health and beauty benefits for brides. For one thing, they keep your skin moist and smooth. In addition, these "good" fats keep your brain functioning, which is important for a bride with many important decisions to make. And they can help ward off stress and depression, also important for brides-to-be.

Good Fats vs. Bad Fats

Use the following list as a reference to increase the "good" fats and decrease the "bad" fats in your diet.

Good Fats

Unsaturated fat: Avocado, olive oil, vegetable oils, fish (salmon, halibut, tuna), raw nuts (walnuts, almonds, cashews), seeds (pumpkin, sunflower, sesame), and flaxseeds

Bad Fats

Saturated fat: Whole milk, cheese, butter, full-fat ice cream, meats, poultry, and tropical oils.

Hydrogenated or trans fat: Most deep-fried foods, margarine, crackers, cookies, pies, and baked goods. Check labels for "hydrogenated" oils in ingredients lists.

Dietary Fats Plan

You still need to eat dietary sources of fat in moderation because they are high in calories. Your goal for total fat intake should be approximately 20–35 percent of the total calories in your diet. Saturated fat ("bad" fat) should be less than 10 percent of your total calories. Reduce the saturated fat in your diet, replace it with unsaturated fat ("good" fat), and avoid trans fat as much as possible. You may need to monitor your fat intake more closely if you have a family history of heart disease or poor cholesterol levels.

Most of the food sources that yield beneficial fats also make good protein sources. Refer to the following section for lists of protein foods and their amount of total fat and saturated fat to help you balance protein and fat in your diet.

Protein Power

Our bodies prefer to use carbohydrates first, then fat, and lastly, protein for energy. Protein performs many other necessary functions in our body. Healthy brides need protein for maintaining muscles, beautiful hair, skin, and teeth. In addition, nutrients in protein help with metabolism, which is the process of digesting carbohydrates, protein, and fat.

It's very common for women to not get enough protein in their diet because they are trying to avoid fat. Protein and fat tend to occur together in food. But, as discussed in the previous section, fats are an essential part of nutrition.

Feeling weak and being prone to illness are signs that you're not getting enough protein. As a healthy bride, you need protein for a healthy immune system and to maintain muscle built in your Healthy Bride workout program. This doesn't mean that you need to down protein-powder drinks and raw eggs to build muscle. You don't need a ton of protein. It all comes down to having the right balance.

If your diet is high in carbohydrates and fats, replace some of those foods with protein foods that are low in saturated fat. This will slow the emptying of the stomach, which will help with weight loss. Protein takes longer for the body to digest, so you don't get the energy highs and lows followed by hunger pangs that you can get from eating a diet lacking adequate protein.

Protein from animal sources include meats (poultry, beef, pork, and fish), eggs, and dairy products. (As stated earlier, dairy products are also high in carbohydrates.) Choose meats that are low in saturated fat, such as chicken and turkey breasts, and lean cuts of beef. When you are buying lunch meats, seek out meats that don't have nitrates and nitrites in them. *Nitrites* and *nitrates* are preservatives that have recently been implicated in having the potential to increase the risk of colon cancer. If you can find a deli with sliced roasted turkey, this is the better whole food choice. And by all means avoid hot dogs and processed meats; they contain the most nitrites or nitrates. Check the ingredient list for sodium nitrate or sodium nitrite, and avoid these products.

Eggs are a good low-calorie, nutritious protein source. The American Heart Association recommends that you limit cholesterol in your diet to 300 mg or less per day. One egg yolk contains 212 mg of cholesterol. This means that you can eat up to one whole egg per day depending on what other cholesterol-containing foods you have that day. Meat and dairy products contain cholesterol that can add up quickly, so you may not want to have an egg every day. To reduce your cholesterol and fat intake when preparing eggs, separate the egg white from the egg yolk because the yolk is where all the cholesterol and fat is. For a low-fat meal, use one whole egg and add egg whites when making an omelet. To err on the side of caution, if you have high cholesterol or an increased risk of heart disease, discuss your egg intake with a dietitian or nutritionist.

The vegetarian sources of protein listed in the Healthy Non-meat Sources of Protein table on page 160 also contain carbohydrates. Usually vegetarian diets aim to be lower in saturated fat. But a vegetarian diet can be high in saturated fat if high-fat dairy products such as cheese are used to replace meat; this is not a good strategy for optimum health or weight loss. Full-fat dairy is high in fat, saturated fat, and calories. For a better balance of healthy low-fat protein, use a combination of non-animal or vegetarian sources of protein such as legumes (beans), nuts, and seeds along with your dairy products unless you are a vegan (vegans are vegetarians that do not eat dairy products). If you would rather not become a full-fledged vegetarian, get the best of both worlds: Eat lean meats, fish, and a variety of vegetarian sources of protein.

Legumes are a superior food because they are low in fat and high in fiber, minerals, B vitamins, and protein. Your body's B vitamins are depleted during times of high stress, so replenishing these vitamins will be very important during the time leading up to your wedding day.

How Much Protein Do You Need?

THE GENERAL RECOMMENDATION for protein is 10–35 percent of the total calories you eat. Here is a simple formula you can use to calculate how many grams of protein you need. Take your weight in pounds and divide it by 2.2 to get your weight in kilograms, then multiply that number by 0.8. Then multiply your weight in kilograms by 1.0. This result (which is 80–100 percent of your weight in kilograms) represents the range of how many grams of protein you need. For example, if you weigh 145 pounds, divide 145 by 2.2; the result is 66 kilograms (rounding up), your weight in kilograms. Multiply 66 by 0.8; the result is 53. Then multiply 66 times 1.0; the result is 66. If you weight 145 pounds, your protein requirements would then be in the range of 53–66 grams per day. You will need a little more protein if you are running marathons or exercising at a high intensity for greater than 60 minutes per day. In that case, multiply your weight in kilograms by 1.2 to find the grams of protein needed.

Type	Percent total fat	Percent saturated fat
Chicken breast, skinless, roasted	19	6
Turkey breast, skinless, roasted	5	2
Turkey, whole, with skin, roasted	30	9
Beef: Top round, eye round, mock-tender steak, shoulder pot roast, round tip, shoulder steak, top sirloin, and bottom round	35 or less	12 or less
Eggs	6	19
Fish*: Salmon (wild Atlantic and Pacific, coho), halibut, and tuna	8–40	6 or less

*The fish listed here are low in saturated fat and excellent sources of essential fats.
Source: USDA Nutrient Database for Standard Reference

Concerns About Seafood

SEAFOOD IS A HEALTHY PART of a balanced diet. Unfortunately, because of environmental pollution and fishing practices, overconsumption of certain types of fish can lead to certain health risks. The table on the following page contains some general guidelines for lowering your chances of exposure to mercury and other contaminates when selecting fish. This is especially important if you are planning on having children. (Pregnant women who consume fish contaminated with mercury have an increased risk of bearing children with neurological disorders.)

Foods contaminated with heavy metals such as mercury and lead, pesticides, PCBs, and other chemicals can cause short-term or long-term health problems and are best avoided or limited in the diet. Your local health department can provide information on the safety of eating locally caught fish.

Find a reputable fishmonger or store to provide the healthiest seafood. Don't be afraid to ask questions. Information on seafood safety is constantly changing as new data becomes available. Use the following websites to stay up to date on these health issues.

• **Center for Food Safety and Consumer Advisory** (www.cfsan.fda.gov/seafood1.html). This site covers health issues and advisories related to eating seafood.

• **U.S. Environmental Protection Agency** (www.epa.gov/waterscience/fish/advisory.html). This site covers health issues and advisories related to eating seafood.

• **Monterey Bay Aquarium** (www.mbayaq.org/cr/seafood-watch.asp). This site covers information on seafood consumption and environmental sustainability issues.

• **Environmentally Responsible Seafood** (www.ecofish.com). This site tells you how to support ecologically sound fisheries and has recipes.

RECOMMENDATIONS FOR SEAFOOD	
Consumption Guidelines	**Types of Fish**
Avoid	Shark, swordfish, king mackerel, tilefish (golden snapper or golden bass)*, and striped bass (wild)**
No more than one 6 oz serving per month**	Salmon (farm-raised/Atlantic) and tuna (albacore)
No more than two 6 oz servings per month	Orange roughy and grouper
No more than three 6 oz servings per month	Sturgeon (wild)
No more than four 6 oz servings per month	Tuna (bluefin)
No more than two 6 oz servings per week*	A combination of canned tuna (light tuna), catfish, pollock, salmon (wild/Pacific), and shrimp

* EPA and FDA recommendations
** Recommendations are for women in their childbearing years
Source: www.pccnaturalmarkets.com/images/issues/seafood/seafoodhealthadvisoryspr04.pdf (PCC Natural Markets, Seafood Health Advisory Chart)

Folate (a B vitamin that's also known as folic acid) is important for wound healing, building muscle, and maintaining a healthy heart. If you plan to get pregnant, folate is important in preventing birth defects. Leafy greens and legumes are good sources of folate.

Find creative ways to incorporate beans into your diet. Throw some garbanzo or kidney beans on a salad, or make soup with black, white, or any other variety of beans, such as chili or lentil soup. Nibble on a garbanzo-bean hummus spread or eat edamame (cooked soybeans) as a snack. Hummus

HEALTHY NON-MEAT SOURCES OF PROTEIN		
Type	Percent of fat	Percent of saturated fat
Legumes (dried beans): Lentils, garbanzos, pintos, kidney beans, and black beans	.06–13	Less than .05
Nuts: Walnuts, almonds, cashews, and pecans	70–80	Less than .1
Seeds: Pumpkin, sunflower, and sesame	36–75	Less than .1
Vegetarian products: Tofu, veggie burgers, gluten, and tempeh	Varies by product, check labels	Varies by product, check labels

(sometimes spelled "hummous") can usually be found in the deli section of the grocery store.

Raw nuts are a good vegetarian source of protein and are not subject to rancidity (which happens when the oil goes bad from exposure to heat and air) the way roasted nuts can be. Stored properly, nuts will maintain their important nutritional qualities. Try to find a good supplier of raw nuts and seeds; find a store that has constant turnover so that you know the nuts haven't been sitting on a shelf or in a bin for a long period of time.

Calcium: Strong Bones for Life

We all know that we need calcium to maintain strong bones. If you are over 35, you have already reached your peak bone mass. Whether you are younger or older than 30–35 years old, adequate calcium is important for both building and maintaining bone mass. Some of the cardio exercises and all the weight-training exercises found in this book will help with bone maintenance. For a total bone maintenance program, it also is key to have a diet of high-calcium foods.

It's a good idea to avoid drinking a lot of soda or to eliminate it completely. Sodas can be high in phosphorus, which can lead to mineral imbalances that cause your body to lose calcium. Similar effects have been seen with high-protein diets. Instead of having a soda, have a glass of nonfat milk, enriched soymilk, or enriched rice milk—all are chock-full of calcium.

Dairy products contain both protein and carbohydrates and are high in calcium. Eat or drink dairy products that are nonfat or low-fat, such as nonfat milk and nonfat or low-fat yogurt, to keep saturated-fat intake down. You also should eat cheese in small amounts because of its high sodium and saturated-fat content. Dairy products are a good source of calcium, but don't forget the nondairy sources as well. Check the Food Sources of Calcium sidebar and Appendix A for both dairy and nondairy sources of calcium.

Remember, getting the right balance of nutrients and eating everything in moderation will keep your bones healthy. Try to get 1,000–1,200 milligrams of calcium a day. Refer to the calcium serving sizes in Appendix A to work toward getting enough calcium in your diet.

If you are finding it difficult to meet your calcium needs through food alone, you should take a daily calcium supplement that includes vitamin D to boost your calcium intake.

Water for the Weary

Last but not least, water is very important. Hydrate for health! Water has many wonderful qualities: It has zero calories, aids the metabolism, and keeps us mentally and physically alert. In my practice, I've seen many brides who have increased their water intake and immediately noticed how much more alert and energetic they felt.

FOOD SOURCES OF CALCIUM	
Food	**Recommendation**
Dairy products: Milk, cheese, and yogurt	Can be high in calories; choose nonfat or low-fat products
Vegetables: Leafy greens (especially kale) and broccoli	Eat plenty of these for their additional nutritional value. (Check out the Leafy Greens Sauté recipe in Appendix B.)
Almonds	Also a good source of unsaturated fat
Enriched rice milk and soymilk	These enriched beverages usually will have the same amount of calcium as cow's milk.

Proper hydration allows all those nutrients to circulate to needed areas in the body. In addition, it helps to detox (or draw impurities from) your system, and it prevents constipation, which is especially important if you're increasing your fiber intake.

Sometimes dehydration can feel deceptively like hunger. Next time you're hungry, drink a big glass of water and see how you feel. Drinking water is a much better solution than drinking caffeinated drinks such as cola, coffee, and tea. These are diuretics and can cause you to lose more water.

Being well hydrated has its aesthetic benefits too. It plumps up your skin, giving it a more youthful appearance with less visible wrinkles.

Set a goal of drinking at least 8–12 eight-ounce glasses of water a day. Don't wait for thirst to tell you to drink water; you are already dehydrated by that time. With your workout program, you will need additional water to replenish the losses from sweating and breathing. This will prevent fatigue and improve your performance. Drink water before, during, and after exercise.

If you currently don't drink much water, slowly ramp up toward your goal and your body will adapt to the increased water intake. If you try to drink too much when your body isn't used to it, you may feel bloated and find yourself frequently running to the bathroom. Our bodies are quite adaptable but they like small changes.

Proceed with Caution: Foods to Avoid or Reduce

This section discusses a few items that may sabotage your Healthy Bride nutrition program, tempting as they may be: sweeteners, alcohol, and caffeine.

Sweeteners

Categorized as carbohydrates, sweeteners provide the most concentrated calories. Avoid white sugar, brown sugar, dextrose sucrose, and high-fructose corn syrup. These are refined sweeteners that have no nutritional value. If using a sweetener, try to use honey, maple syrup, molasses, brown-rice syrup, or dehydrated cane juice instead because they are less processed. Even so, use them sparingly.

Don't believe the hype surrounding artificial sweeteners such as aspartame (Equal, NutraSweet), saccharine (Sweet'N Low), and acesulfame-K. There is little evidence that artificial sweeteners help with weight loss. Those who use artificial sweeteners tend to make up the calories or consume more because they feel less satisfied. If you have a sweet tooth, use the less-processed sweeteners, which provide calories and will give you some satisfaction. Use the real stuff; enjoy it, but only in small amounts.

Alcoholic Drinks

With all the celebrations surrounding your wedding, alcohol may be abundant. If you decide to drink alcohol, do so in moderation. For the bride, and women in general, moderation is defined as one drink per day. (Moderation

The Importance of Fiber

MOST AMERICANS don't get enough fiber in their diet because they don't eat enough whole grains, legumes (beans), fruits, and vegetables. Soluble fiber can help to lower cholesterol and absorb fat in the diet so that what you eat doesn't deposit as fat on your body. Soluble fiber can be found in legumes, oats, and fruit.

What you may not realize is that *fiber is the secret ingredient to weight loss.* All high-fiber foods are low in calories. They make you feel full, keep your colon healthy, and prevent constipation. (FYI, if you're not having daily bowel movements, you definitely need more fiber in your diet.)

The best time to get a jump-start on your fiber consumption is during breakfast—after all, it is the most important meal of the day. Have a whole-grain cereal with some fruit in the morning. Then incorporate legumes into your daily diet. This will help you meet your fiber goals easily.

Work toward a goal of at least 20–25 grams of fiber per day. If your diet is currently low in fiber, gradually increase the amount of fiber you eat and the amount of water you drink to allow your body to adapt. If you try to increase fiber in your diet too quickly, you may run into constipation problems (just what you are trying to prevent). Also make sure you do increase your water intake at the same time. Become a "regular" bride; your digestive system will thank you.

for men is two drinks per day.) If a woman drinks more than one drink per day, the protective effects of alcohol against heart disease are greatly reduced. One drink amounts to 12 ounces of beer, 5 ounces of wine (at 12 percent alcohol), or 1.5 ounces of 80-proof distilled spirits.

If you don't drink alcohol, there's really no reason to start. Alcohol has many empty calories that can add up fast. A glass of celebratory champagne can add up to 193 calories; red or white wine, 130–150 calories; and beer, 150–220 calories. Mixed drinks can range from 150–1,000 calories depending on the type.

You also should avoid alcoholic beverages if any of the following apply:

- You will be driving or taking part in an activity that requires skill or coordination.

- You are taking medications that may interact with the alcohol. (Ask your physician or pharmacist if you are not sure.)

- You cannot restrict your alcohol intake.

- You have medical conditions that require abstention from alcohol.

- You are pregnant.

If you are unsure about whether you should drink alcoholic beverages because of health or other reasons, consult your health-care professional.

Caffeinated Beverages

I hope you'll have so much additional energy from the Healthy Bride work-out and nutrition program that you won't need any caffeine. Drinking caffeinated beverages such as coffee and colas can make you feel more tired by giving you a quick boost of energy followed by a bigger slump. It is especially important to avoid drinking caffeinated beverages if you are susceptible to irritability, anxiety, or stress. Being a bride-to-be is a stressful time. Don't let caffeine increase your stress, burn you out, and leave you in an extended energy slump. Caffeine can also affect your quality of sleep. Brides don't need (or want) dark circles under their eyes.

Mixed caffeinated coffee drinks that include sweeteners, flavorings, and cream can provide a huge amount of fat and calories that can add extra pounds very quickly. Want more proof? Check out the Starbucks website (www.starbucks.com/retail/nutrition_info.asp) for nutritional information on the company's various coffee drinks. A grande whole-milk Caffe Mocha with whipped cream adds up to a whopping 430 calories at 47 percent fat. Think about the balanced meal you could have at that calorie level instead.

Numerous brides have told me, "Please don't take away my coffee!" (I realize giving up coffee may be a tough sell.) If you need your coffee, try to limit it to one cup a day in the morning. But try not to overdo any caffeine.

A healthy alternative to coffee is green tea; it has some caffeine and high levels of antioxidants. You may want to use green tea to wean yourself off coffee. It's easier to transition from coffee to green tea than to give up caffeine altogether. You may even decrease breast-cancer risk by drinking green tea.

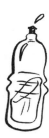

CHAPTER 15

Keep a Well-stocked Kitchen

Having a well-stocked kitchen allows you to make healthy meals in a pinch. Having staple foods on hand that store well helps you develop a repertoire of quick meals, which can be economical and "waist-saving." A well-stocked kitchen doesn't mean you have to endure a refrigerator bin full of rotting vegetables. A little planning goes a long way.

As part of my practice, I take brides on grocery-store tours. We may go to their usual store, or we may go to a new store that they have felt intimidated by. This tour gives them a new perspective on shopping and increases their awareness of new foods. If you're like most people, you hurriedly dash into your regular store, grab your usual items (along with a few impulse items from the ends of the aisles), and go. People have a tendency to buy the same foods repeatedly and not take the time to explore new or different foods. How often do you take a whole hour just looking at various foods and reading labels?

Decipher Food Labels

Before your next shopping trip, learn how to read food labels. Go into your kitchen and grab a box of cereal, can of soup, or packaged meal. Don't get caught up in the advertising on the label. Labels that claim what's inside is "low-fat," "no cholesterol," and "low-carb" don't really tell you much

Nutrition Facts	
Serving Size: 1 cup (244g)	
Servings 4	
Amount Per Serving	
Calories 120	Calories from Fat 40
	% Daily Value*
Total Fat 4.5g	8%
Saturated Fat 3g	15%
Cholesterol 20mg	6%
Sodium 120mg	6%
Total Carbohydrate 12g	4%
Dietary Fiber 0g	0%
Sugars 12g	
Protein 8g	
Vitamin A 10% ▪	Vitamin C 4%
Calcium 30% ▪	Iron 0%
*Percent Daily Values are based on a 2,000 calorie diet.	

and are not regulated as stringently. Manufacturers can put almost anything on the packaging, whether it is 100 percent truthful or not.

Focus on the nutrition facts panel and ingredients list, which are strictly regulated. All packaged foods must have both. The sample nutrition facts panel on the previous page is for a quart of 2% fat milk. Here are some basic guidelines for interpreting the nutrition facts panel:

- **Serving size and servings per container.** The serving size is the measurement of food that the nutritional information is based upon. The sample label shows a serving size of 1 cup and that the container consists of "four servings." This doesn't mean you have to eat or drink this specific amount (1 cup) per meal or snack. Some manufacturers will list small serving sizes to make the product appear lower in calorie content. See if the serving size is equivalent to what you will eat or drink and then see how the numbers add up.

- **Calories.** This indicates the total calories per serving (in this label's case, 120 calories). Remember, if the package contains two servings and you eat or drink the whole package, your calories will be doubled.

- **Calories from fat.** This is the number of calories that come from fat. Divide this number by calories per serving to get the percentage of fat per serving. For example, 40 calories from fat divided by 120 calories equals 33% fat. (Bet you didn't know 2% milk is actually 33% fat.) Aim for: Less than 20–35% fat for total calories per day.

Mysteries Revealed in the List of Ingredients

THE WRITING CAN BE so small on some product labels that you feel the need for a magnifying glass to find out what is in your food. Reading ingredients lists may inspire plenty of "ah-ha" moments, such as my discovery that some canned beans have sugar added to them.

Keep in mind that ingredients are presented in descending order on food labels, from highest amount of content to lowest. Reading an ingredients list can be very enlightening. For example, I once noticed that a particular package of tortillas marked as "whole-wheat tortillas" actually contained very little whole wheat. If the tortillas were truly whole wheat, something like "whole-wheat flour" would have appeared at the beginning of the ingredients list. Here's another example: On a grocery-store tour, one of the brides I've worked with discovered that her favorite cereal had artificial sweetener along with refined sweeteners in it. She opted to change cereals because

she didn't want to keep artificial sweeteners in her diet. In addition, scouring the ingredients of the foods you eat is a good way to weed out hydrogenated fats—the "bad" fats discussed earlier—from your diet.

To determine whether a food item is a whole-grain product, look for the words "whole wheat," "whole grain," or "brown-rice flour" at or near the beginning of the list. If the label says "wheat flour," "unbleached wheat flour," "enriched wheat flour," or "rice flour," you are holding a refined grain product and not a whole food.

Now that you have a better understanding of how to read food labels, try pretending you're at the library next time you go the grocery store. Wander through the aisles and look at the labels, and read the nutrition facts panel and the ingredients list. Know what is in the food you're buying. Remember, the food industry counts on your lack of attention to hook you on unhealthy tastes and flavors.

• **Percent daily value.** This is how much a serving will contribute to your total daily intake of food. These amounts usually appear in the nutrition facts panel under the heading "% Daily Value." (Because percent

Nutritional Goals for Total Calories

THE FOLLOWING ARE the ideal nutritional percentage goals for carbohydrates, protein, and total fat, which are supported by the American Dietetic Association (ADA):

Carbohydrates: 45–65%

Protein: 10–35%

Total fat: Less than 20–35%

To calculate calories for protein, carbohydrates, and fat:

* *Each gram of protein or carbohydrates equals 4 calories (multiply 1 gram of protein or carbohydrate by 4).*

* *Each gram of fat is equal to 9 calories (multiply 1 gram of fat by 9).*

daily value is standardized for a 2,000-calorie diet, your needs may be higher or lower.) These numbers provide a rough estimate of how this food fits into your total intake for the day. For example, if sodium is marked as 50% of the daily value on the food label, this means it is 50% (or 1,150 milligrams) of the 2,300 milligrams or less recommended for the day. If this serving accounts for one meal or snack that day, it's too high in sodium. Considering that you will be eating two other meals and snacks on any given day, this amount would take you well over the daily limit for sodium. In some cases, such as with fiber, it's OK to exceed the percent daily value. For now, it may be easier to focus on the numbers for total fat, fiber, and sugar instead of using the percent daily value as the primary guideline for your daily food intake.

- **Total fat.** This represents the number of grams of fat per serving. If "calories from fat" (an optional field) is not listed on your food label, multiply the number right after "total fat" (in this case, 4.5) by 9 (number of calories per gram of fat) to figure out the calories from fat per serving. You may not see subcategories for total fat depending what the product is. If the nutrition facts panel contains subcategories, saturated, trans, monounsaturated, and polyunsaturated fat may be listed. Multiply the saturated fat by 9, and divide the result by the total calories per serving to figure out the percentage of saturated fat. *Aim for:* Less than 10% saturated fat for total calories per day.

- **Sodium.** This represents the milligrams of sodium per serving. *Aim for:* Less than 2,300 milligrams per day.

- **Fiber.** This represents the amount of fiber per serving. *Aim for:* At least 20–25 grams per day.

- **Sugar.** This represents the grams of sugar per serving. Some products (such as milk) have naturally occurring sugars, which can make the sugar amount appear high; check the ingredients list for added sugar. Visualize it this way: 12.5 grams of sugar equals one tablespoon. Ask yourself if the amount of sugar seems reasonable and what types of sugar appear on the ingredients list.

To sum up, you should pay closest attention to the serving size, number of calories, calories from total fat along with saturated fat, grams of fiber, and grams of sugar. To access more detailed information about reading food labels, check out the U.S. Food and Drug Administration's website at www. cfsan.fda.gov/~dms/foodlab.html.

Produce Shopping

The produce section is where you should spend most of your shopping time. Thoroughly explore this section. You know those green, leafy vegetables that you're unsure how to prepare? I'm not just talking about spinach. There's kale, chard, Asian greens (such as bok choy and choi sum), and collard greens, too. The Leafy Greens Sauté recipe on page 241 is a quick and easy way to prepare these types of vegetables. Also check out the recommended cookbooks listed at the end of Chapter 18.

Go for a range of color in produce. Any fruit or vegetable with rich colors tends to be rich in antioxidants. Antioxidants prevent cellular damage that can lead to cancer and heart disease. They may even slow aging. Choose red, green, yellow, and orange bell peppers; tomatoes; berries; and oranges. Eat from a rainbow of colors to get a mix of antioxidants. You can hardly go wrong in the produce section, so pick a variety of fruits and vegetables. Choose seasonal fruits and vegetables because they have a higher nutritional value, taste better, and are more economical. Bear in mind, these foods are perishable, so only buy what you can consume within three to five days.

A Staple Food Shopping List

As a busy bride-to-be, you don't have a lot of time to be running to the grocery store every few days. Following is a shopping list of staple items that you can store for longer periods of time and are good to have available in the kitchen for quick meals. Continue to use these ideas as you set up your kitchen with your new husband.

Protein Items

As part of a well-balanced diet, protein helps to stave off hunger and provides necessary nutrients for maintaining muscles, healthy skin, and hair.

- **Canned beans.** Be sure to check the ingredients list to see that no sugar has been added. Also, be careful with sodium levels. *Potential uses*: Salads, quick chili, soups, casseroles, and bean spreads.

- **Canned vegetarian or low-fat refried beans.** Again, check the ingredients list and watch out for sodium levels. Don't buy products that contain lard or hydrogenated oils (trans fat). *Potential uses*: Quesadillas, tacos, and burritos.

- **Dried legumes (beans).** You'll have to plan ahead to cook these. Soak large beans (such as kidney, pinto, black, and garbanzo) overnight and drain the soaking water and add fresh water before cooking. Smaller beans such as lentils don't need to be soaked overnight before cooking. Depending on the type of bean, soaked beans can take 30-60 minutes to cook. Dried beans store well, for those days when it's too cold or rainy to go to the store. *Potential uses:* Soups, salads, casseroles, main dishes, and chili.

- **Edamame (soybeans).** These can be found in the frozen food section. Store them at home in the freezer and reheat as needed. *Potential uses:* High-protein snack, in stir-fries, and salads.

Dairy Products Shopping

DAIRY PRODUCTS are a good source of calcium. They also can be high in saturated fat, so choose low-fat and nonfat varieties when making your selection. Dairy products such as cheese and milk should be bought on an "as needed" basis since they tend to spoil within a week or two. Some dairy products last longer than others; check for expiration dates and plan accordingly. Yogurt tends to keep longer— about two to three weeks—and may be part of the staples that you keep on hand. Store all dairy products in the refrigerator.

- **Nuts.** Buy raw nuts (such as walnuts, almonds, and cashews) and store them in an airtight container in the refrigerator or freezer to preserve the natural oils. You can roast small amounts as needed. To roast nuts or seeds, preheat the oven to 300°F, spread the nuts or seeds on a baking sheet, and bake for approximately 8–12 minutes while tossing frequently to roast all sides. *Potential uses:* Snacks, in breakfast cereals, in salads, and stir-fries.

- **Nut butters (such as peanut, cashew, and almond).** Use natural nut butters without added sugar or fats, especially hydrogenated fat. Store in the refrigerator to preserve the oils. You may need to stir the nut butter before using if the oils have separated. *Potential uses:* Spread on toast or sandwiches, and eat as a snack (on whole-grain crackers or apples).

- **Seed butters (such as tahini, sesame-seed butter, and pumpkin-seed butter).** Store in the refrigerator. Pumpkin-seed butter is a fairly new product and may not be widely available. *Potential uses:* Spread on toast or sandwiches, eat as a snack, and use in noodle sauces.

- **Eggs.** This protein staple keeps fresh up to one month when stored in a carton or covered container in the refrigerator. Hard-boiled eggs will keep for one week in the refrigerator. *Potential uses:* Add to fried rice (stir-fried, not deep fried), eat as a meal or snack (poached or hard-boiled), add to salads, and make omelets and frittatas.

- **Canned tuna and/or canned salmon.** Review the Concerns About Seafood sidebar (page 158) if you plan to limit your consumption of canned tuna. *Potential uses:* On sandwiches, on top of salad greens, in casseroles, and in spreads.

- **Frozen fish.** Avoid breaded fish sticks! They usually contain trans fat and other unhealthy ingredients. Buy plain frozen-fish fillets such as wild salmon and halibut and prepare to your taste. *Potential uses:* As part of a balanced meal with a whole-grain carbohydrate, on fish tacos, and on salads.

- **Lean meat.** This can be bought frozen or fresh and then frozen until ready to use. See the Protein Power section and the table "Healthy Non-meat Sources of

Protein" on page 160 for a list of low-fat meats. Chicken and turkey breast are lowest in fat. These can be found pre-ground as a healthy substitute to hamburger meat. *Potential uses:* Add to spaghetti sauces, tacos, salads, stir-fries, and casseroles.

More Vegetables

Vegetables are good sources of fiber and antioxidants, and are good for colon health and disease prevention.

- **Salad greens.** This is not exactly a nonperishable item, but it's worth preparing for a week's worth of salads. Select red-leaf, green-leaf, or romaine lettuce. Rinse and then dry in a salad spinner. Your personally prepared salad will last longer than the store-bought salad mixes when stored in a Ziploc bag or other airtight container. Depending on the freshness of the greens used, they can last for more than five days in the refrigerator. The store-bought salad mixes will do in a pinch, but don't expect them to last more than a few days. See the Colorful Tossed Salad recipe on page 244 for salad ingredients and topping ideas. *Potential uses:* Add protein for a complete meal, or eat as a side dish to a balanced meal.

- **Frozen vegetables.** Avoid the vegetable combinations that contain mostly starchy vegetables, such as carrots, potatoes, and peas, or ones that have added fat. These will be higher in calories. Many frozen stir-fry mixes will have a better variety of lower calorie vegetables, such as broccoli, snow peas, and bean sprouts. Or buy the individual packages of frozen broccoli or spinach. *Potential uses:* Soups, stir-fries, and side vegetable dishes.

Carbohydrate Items

Carbohydrates are our primary energy source. The whole-grain foods listed are rich in fiber, vitamins, and minerals. The colorful berries are excellent sources of antioxidants.

- **Whole-wheat pasta or brown-rice pasta.** Check the ingredients list to make sure the manufacturer is being truthful in calling the product "whole grain." See if whole wheat or brown rice is the first or only ingredient listed. Also, when cooking and eating pasta, don't overdo it on the portions. Watch your portion size very carefully; pasta calories can add up fast. *Potential uses:* Main course and pasta salads with protein and vegetables.

- **Corn or whole-wheat tortillas.** Check the ingredients list and avoid any made with lard (animal fat) or hydrogenated fats. Is corn or whole wheat first on the ingredients list? Store in the freezer until you're ready to use them. *Potential uses:* Quesadillas, tacos, and burritos.

- **Brown rice.** I strongly recommend you invest in a rice cooker; you won't regret it. With a rice cooker, you just add water, push the button, and *voila*—the rice is cooked! Store extra cooked rice in an airtight container in the refrigerator for up to three days. Add a little water to reheat. *Potential uses:* Stir-fried rice, in soup, part of a balanced meal with protein and vegetables, serve with a vegetable and protein stir-fry.

- **Oatmeal (rolled or steel cut).** Oatmeal is a great hot breakfast meal that's high in fiber. Rolled oats require a shorter cooking time than steel-cut oats. *Potential uses:* Baked goods and breakfast cereal (add fruit and nuts).

- **Other grains, such as quinoa, amaranth, and millet.** These grains can usually be found in the bulk-food area at a natural-food store. You also may find them packaged in other stores. *Potential uses:* Hot cereals (see Appendix B for sample recipes), grain salads, and as a rice or starch replacement.

- **Frozen berries.** Buy blueberries, raspberries, boysenberries, marionberries, and strawberries, and you'll be rewarded with plenty of colorful antioxidants! *Potential uses:* Smoothies, topping for yogurt, with breakfast cereals, and filling for whole-grain muffins. (See the Wholesome Blueberry Muffins recipe on page 242.)

Other Staples

These foods will round out your meals with additional flavor and variety.

- **Vegetable and/or chicken broth.** You'll find these sold in cans or aseptic boxes (larger sized). *Potential uses:* In stir-fries, pasta dishes, and soups.

- **Meatless spaghetti sauces.** Check the ingredients list for added cheese or excess oil, which can rack up the calories. Add beans for a vegetarian protein source. *Potential uses:* With a pasta main course or side dish, and as a pour over baked chicken breast for a quick chicken cacciatore.

- **Canned tomatoes.** You can use a can of tomatoes to add plenty of flavor to dishes, without the additional salt. *Potential uses*: Soups, sauces, casseroles, and stews.

- **Salsa.** You can find fresh salsa in the refrigerated section of your grocery store or in jars on the shelves; the latter will keep longer. Most salsas are low in fat. Some varieties have the bonus of added vegetables, such as corn and beans. *Potential uses:* On quesadillas, tacos, burritos, and salads; also try adding vinegar to create a nonfat, low-calorie salad dressing.

- **Olive oil.** This is a good source of monounsaturated fat. Do not use olive oil for high-heat cooking; instead use organic canola oil or safflower oil. *Potential uses:* Salad dressing, cooking, sautéing, and stir-fries.

CHAPTER 16

Create Meal Plans

Meal plans can help you stay on track with healthy foods. This section gives you the freedom to choose foods and recipes that fit your food preferences and lifestyle. With the information you've learned in the nutrition section of this book, you can create your own balanced and healthy meal plans. Sample meal plans can be found at the end of this chapter.

Use the following instructions to guide you in meal planning:

1. **Review.** Familiarize yourself with the balanced food pyramid and serving sizes listed in Appendix A. This will give you an overview of portion sizes and food groups to incorporate into your daily menu.

2. **Food lists.** Create a list of your favorite foods and recipes. Incorporate some new foods or recipes that you are willing to try. Divide these foods and recipes into the various food categories. Use the foods listed in the Anatomy of a Healthy Diet (Chapter 14) and the section A Staple Food Shopping List on page 172 for basic ideas. Refer to the recipes in Appendix B and the referenced cookbooks at the end of this section for new ideas. Make creating a collection of foods and recipes your own little research project.

3. **Healthy foods.** Are you unsure about whether a food or recipe is healthy? Most recipes will have nutritional information listed. Use the Decipher Food Labels section on page 167 to understand the nutritional breakdown. If a recipe doesn't have the nutritional information, use the knowledge that you've gained in this part of the book to examine the ingredients. Are they high in fat? Refined? Dense in calories and not nutrients? Whole foods–based? With experience, you'll be able to modify recipes to make them healthier. To find information about a specific food or ingredient not listed in this book, you can use the USDA National Nutrient Database online at www.nal.usda.gov/fnic/foodcomp/search/ to look up its nutritional breakdown. See the following chapter for a detailed explanation of how to use the database.

4. **Meal plan.** Assemble your food and recipes list into three meals and two snacks for each day. Then ask yourself if they fit into your lifestyle. Be realistic about how often you will cook or take your lunch to work. You may need to create plans that include eating take-out food or dining out. See the Dining Out: Tips to Guide You through the Menu section on page 136 for help in selecting these types of foods. In creating your meal plan, try to have some protein with each meal and, optimally, try to have some protein with each snack.

5. **Portion sizes.** Refer to the recommended serving sizes in Appendix A to determine the number of servings to aim for in each food group. This will help you decide how to proportion and distribute the food for the day. Use the Nutritional Goals for Total Calories sidebar on page 170 for details on how to distribute the protein, carbohydrates, and fat in a meal.

6. **Grocery list.** Once you have created a meal plan, you can easily create your grocery list and stock your kitchen.

This process may seem tedious at first, but with practice it will become more natural.

Sample Meal Plans

Here are some samples of daily meal plans you can follow for well-balanced meals and snacks. Recipes for some of these foods may be found in Appendix B. Remember to drink 8–12 glasses of water per day as well.

Sample Meal Plan I

Breakfast: Bowl of oatmeal with walnuts, blueberries, skim milk, and maple syrup

Snack: Apple with peanut butter

Lunch: Roasted turkey breast sandwich on whole-grain bread with lettuce, tomatoes, and bell peppers, and a cup of vegetable and bean soup

Snack: Nonfat fruit yogurt with nuts and granola

Dinner: Baked chicken breast, steamed broccoli, whole-wheat roll, and green salad with sliced pears

Sample Meal Plan 2

Breakfast: Bowl of cereal (Oat and Millet with Fruit) with cashews, skim milk, and maple syrup

Snack: Banana and handful of walnuts

Lunch: Garbanzo Bean and Quinoa Salad on a bed of mixed greens

Snack: Carrots and celery with hummus spread

Dinner: Lemon Ginger Salmon, Leafy Greens Sauté, brown basmati rice, and Colorful Tossed Salad

Sample Meal Plan 3

Breakfast: Energizing Fruit Smoothie and a small handful of almonds

Snack: Wholesome Blueberry Muffin

Lunch: Colorful Tossed Salad with canned tuna

Snack: Pear and edamame (soybeans)

Dinner: Vegetarian black bean chili, corn tortillas, and a mixed green salad

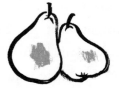

CHAPTER 17

Track Your Progress

Recording your food intake is critical to making changes in your nutritional habits. To make a positive change, you need to see where you are starting from. Then you can determine where the improvements will be made. Food journaling gives you a baseline to work with.

Keeping a food journal is admittedly difficult to do consistently, despite the many benefits. Yes, it does take time and commitment to write down your food intake. However, no one else is looking over your shoulder, so you can honestly evaluate your current nutritional habits. Invest a few minutes each day to write down what foods you eat. This will provide valuable insight into your eating behaviors. People who use food journals have the most success in changing eating habits and managing their weight.

Start by making copies of the sample daily food journal on page 187. You can reduce the size to carry it in your purse. Record within two hours of eating so that you don't forget what you ate that day. (It's amazing how our selective memory can work.) Start by recording what you eat a few days a week. At the end of each week, review your food intake. You may quickly discover you've improved your diet because you had to write it down.

Recognize Your Eating Behaviors

Next, record more days, even those "bad" days on which you know you aren't eating well-balanced meals and snacks. This is hard, but remember that only you will see the entries. Be sure to write down the events of the day, how you were feeling, and how hungry you were so that you can review these details

Elements of Successful Food Journaling

THE FOLLOWING STEPS will help you keep a successful food journal. Note: Each journal page is intended for one day of recorded food intake.

- Write down foods eaten within two hours of consumption.

- Fill in the fields completely, including the time you ate and your degree of hunger, from zero to four (zero means not hungry, four means very hungry). Note serving sizes accurately, along with events, locations, emotions, and physical symptoms at the time of eating.

- Use tick marks to record glasses of water, fruit servings, and vegetable servings. You'll soon find out how good you are at determining serving sizes.

- Assess your journal without judgment—look for patterns, areas for improvement, and any physical or emotional triggers.

- Set small goals that are attainable.

- Don't lose focus on the positive results. Acknowledge them, and move on to the next goal.

at the end of the week. After a while, you'll start to see patterns.

For example, say your mother-in-law wanted the bridesmaids' dresses to be lime green and you ate a whole container of cookie-dough ice cream (not that I'm putting down your mother-in-law or lime-green dresses). Writing this information in your journal and reviewing it later may help you realize that stressful situations can lead you to junk food. As you continue recording and reviewing what you have written, you will begin to see patterns or triggers. Then you can work to develop strategies for changing them.

Evaluate other ways you could have dealt with a particular stressful situation without being self-destructive or judgmental. Instead of using food to make you feel better, channel that energy in a positive way; maybe you could have gone for a run, done a few additional crunches, or cleaned your house to relieve the frustration. Always ask yourself why you are eating, especially when you're not really fulfilling a physical need such as hunger.

Measure Your Success

Next use your journal to look at the foods you ate during the past week or several weeks. Did you accurately record your serving sizes? We have a tendency to underestimate our serving sizes, which can add up to additional calories. Did you set a goal for number of glasses of water, fruit servings, and vegetable servings? Did you meet your goals? If not, maybe you need to set smaller goals. For example, address the water intake for the first month. Then add one additional vegetable or fruit serving per day during the following month. Setting smaller goals allows you to meet long-term goals with less frustration and more reward.

Also, don't forget to acknowledge the positive. If you met a goal, congratulate yourself and reward yourself with something that's not food related. Buy yourself a small gift or pamper yourself with a long, hot bath. If you didn't meet a goal, reevaluate it without judgment—maybe your goal was too high. Set your sights lower and don't give up.

Once you meet your goals for water intake and vegetable and fruit servings, take it to the next level. If you're into numbers, track your intake of protein, fat, carbohydrates, and fiber. There are many websites that provide the nutrient breakdown of various foods. The most accurate and dependable is the USDA National Nutrient Database at www.nal.usda.gov/fnic/foodcomp/search/. To use this site, enter a keyword for the food you want to search on, and then follow the screen prompts for food type and serving size to receive a nutrient breakdown for that food. You'll find a list of calories, vitamins, minerals, protein, fats, and carbohydrates for that food item. Another option to track your daily nutrients and calories is the USDA My Pyramid Tracker at www.mypyramidtracker.gov. You'll need to sign up to use it. Enter your food and serving sizes for the day to receive information on the number of calories and nutrients, and to see if you met the dietary guideline recommendations.

SAMPLE FOOD JOURNAL

Time (a.m./p.m.)	Degree of Hunger (0–4)	Amount	Foods/ Beverages	Locations/ Events	Calories	Protein	Cholesterol	Fat	Fiber
				TOTAL					
				Percentage of Daily Intake					

USE TICK MARKS TO INDICATE YOUR WATER, VEGETABLE, AND FRUIT INTAKE:

Water intake (for each 8 oz glass) ○ ○ ○ ○ ○ ○ ○ ○

Vegetable servings ○ ○ ○ ○ ○

Fruit servings ○ ○ ○ ○ ○

COMMENTS (emotions, physical symptoms, other):

187

CHAPTER 18

Foods for Forever After

If you are not very experienced in the kitchen, don't be afraid to experiment with simple recipes. Everyone is a beginner at some time. There will be failures and successes. Don't put yourself down as a "bad cook" because of one or more failures. Chock it up to a learning experience. Allow yourself time to develop your cooking abilities. Cooking can be satisfying and relaxing. Hopefully you can get your fiancé involved too.

Refer to the recipes in Appendix B as a start. In addition, I encourage you to explore a variety of foods. If you don't know what to do with a new food, get yourself a good cookbook that describes how to prepare it. Try new cookbooks regularly and read cookbooks for ideas. The library can be a good resource if you don't have the space or money for a lot of cookbooks. Dietary change is an ongoing process as you develop new tastes for healthy foods. There's a whole world of new foods to try; don't allow yourself to fall into "food ruts" and eat yourself into boredom.

Making positive nutrition change is an ongoing process of discovery. Don't be discouraged if you have setbacks—you have the rest of your life to work on better nutrition with your future husband. Food provides more than nourishment; it is what brings us together and bonds us spiritually. Use this time to explore and create new food traditions with your new family.

Further Reading

Here are a few fantastic books on choosing foods and preparing them. Use them in good health.

Recommended cookbooks:

- *Vegetarian Cooking for Everyone,* by Deborah Madison (New York, NY: Broadway Books, 1997). This award-winning book is not just a great recipe book, but also an excellent reference book on cooking equipment, basic cooking, and cutting methods. Best of all, it describes a variety of vegetables and how to prepare them.

- *Feeding the Whole Family: Whole Foods Recipes for Babies, Young Children, and Their Parents*, by Cynthia Lair (Seattle, WA: Moon Smile Press, 1998). This is a great introductory book to whole foods. This book offers guidance on how to cook a variety of legumes and whole grains. It contains a great selection of recipes.

- *Greens Glorious Greens! More than 140 Ways to Prepare All Those Great-Tasting, Super-Healthy, Beautiful Leafy Greens,* by Johnna Albi and Catherine Walthers (New York, NY: St. Martin's Press, 1996). This cookbook describes and provides recipes for all the leafy greens and Asian greens that you may have avoided in the grocery store. With this book, you can learn how to incorporate these nutritious greens into your diet in a delicious way.

Recommended books about nutrition and trying new foods:

- *Eat, Drink, and Be Healthy: The Harvard Medical School Guide to Healthy Eating,* by Walter C. Willet, M.D. (New York, NY: Fireside, 2002). This is a good reference for basic nutritional information based on sound research. Use this book to make sense of all the nutritional information that you would normally get through the media.

- *The Visual Food Encyclopedia: The Definitive Practical Guide to Food and Cooking,* edited by François Fortin (New York, NY: Macmillan, 1996). If you are a person who prefers visual instruction, this is the book for you. Expand your world of food with this illustrated book that describes common and uncommon fruits, vegetables, grains, meats, seafood, nuts, seeds, oils, spices, and dairy products. If you ever want to know more about a particular whole food, you can look it up here. This book includes information on nutrition, storage, selection, preparation, and serving ideas.

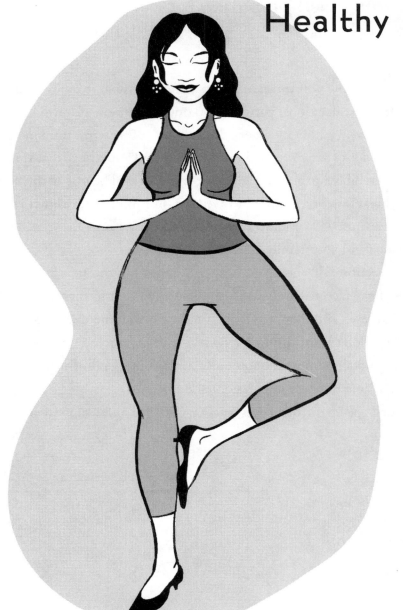

Part Four

Stress and the Healthy Bride

Stress—it's the one thing no bride can hide from when preparing for her wedding day.

S o how will you remain sane, calm, and able to enjoy all the showers, decisions, parties, workouts, decisions, plans, schedules, in-laws, family members, deciswions . . . Phew, just thinking about all the pre-wedding activity makes me stressed out! You know that this process will be incredibly fun at times and your wedding will be one of the best times in your life. However, the road to wedded bliss most assuredly will be paved with bumps and will certainly create some stress not only for you, but also for your fiancé and your family.

This section will show you how to smooth out those bumps as much as possible. Let's face it—we've all seen brides who have turned these bumps into mountains, and they're still recovering from all the drama long after the wedding. I don't want this to happen to you. I want you to be able to cope with any and all bumps and come out at the other end of that road relaxed, rested, and able to enjoy your wedding day.

Before we begin our stress busting, let's see how stressed out you are today.

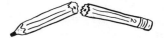

CHAPTER 19

How Stressed Are You?

Bridal Stress Test

Answer the following questions with True or False:

1. I am getting plenty of sleep and I am sleeping well.

   True False

2. I am eating enough and not too much, and I am eating mostly the right things. **True False**

3. I do not find myself ruminating on topics that are bothering me. **True False**

4. I am able to make decisions and feel good about them. **True False**

5. My family is supportive and helpful when it comes to my wedding. **True False**

6. My friends and bridesmaids are supportive and helpful when it comes to my wedding. **True False**

7. My fiancé is sharing in our wedding planning process. **True False**

8. I have time to do most of the things I want to do for my wedding and for myself right now. **True False**

9. My wedding planning is not adversely affecting my job or my friendships. **True False**

10. I feel good about how my wedding day is going to turn out. **True False**

Results

If you answered False to 0–3 questions: You are doing quite well, and there's no need to worry, at least for right now.

If you answered False to 3–6 questions: You are becoming fairly stressed and probably should reevaluate how you are coping with the pressure.

If you answered False to 7–10 questions: We need to talk! Things could be going a lot better for you. Keep reading this section; you really need to de-stress.

If you are not feeling stressed at the moment, great! Keep checking in with yourself. Or come back and take this test from time to time, perhaps once a month until the month of your wedding, and then one time a week during the month of your wedding. The first key to coping with your stress is recognizing that you are stressed and to what degree.

For those of you who answered False to four or more questions on this stress test, help is on the way. There are many ways to release stress. The following pages present a smorgasbord of these techniques, not a set menu. I suggest you read through all the activities in this section first and then select those you think will work best for you. Remember, the higher your score was on this stress test, the more de-stressing you probably require.

Create a Stress Survival Kit

When angry, count ten before you speak; if very angry, one hundred.

—Thomas Jefferson

I heard a story recently about a bride who was so upset with her maid of honor for being 10 minutes late to the rehearsal dinner, she "fired" her right then and there in front of everyone. The truth was that the maid of honor had been downstairs setting up a slideshow she'd made of the bride and her fiancé to show later that night. Had this bride counted to 10 and asked her maid of honor why she was late, there would have been a lot less stress for everyone.

It's so easy to get wound up over the small things that bother us and to lose sight of the bigger picture. And these blowups are the sort of things one never forgets. Will that bride ever forget firing her maid of honor? I'm sure the memory will be with her forever, though it's not exactly one she'd want to keep.

How do you deal with your stress during one of the biggest moments of your life? There's a lot of pressure on you when planning and having your wedding. No question about it. It's how you deal with the stress that counts. One of my favorite sayings is, "It's not what happens to you in life that matters, it's how you deal with what happens to you in life that really makes the difference."

Take some time out and think of the things that make you feel happy, calm, and centered. It might be a certain phrase, a poem, a picture, or a letter you received from a loved one. Or it may be activities, such as taking a deep breath or doing simple yoga moves or meditation. Or it may be something less tangible, such as a smell or a memory from another time. Whatever beacon of calm you choose, make sure it's easy to memorize or carry with you. Any time you feel like you're at the point of "losing it," you will have these soothing memories, icons, quotations, or activities to turn to. Let's call this calming touchstone your "Bridal Stress Survival Kit."

Determine what your survival kit will contain and how you can keep it with you for easy access. When you feel yourself getting stressed, all you need to do is "pull out your kit" and use it. You may have to excuse yourself from some situations (even public ones) for a few minutes, and that is perfectly fine. Do what you need to do to manage the rough spots so that you can keep your wedding-planning process fun.

Simple Ways to Handle Stress

Many books, articles, and websites offer pages and pages of advice on how to deal with stress, and I am sure everyone you could ask will have a perspective on what stress-busting techniques have worked for them. Getting advice is great, but you are on your own path and therefore must create your own program for managing your own stress.

Because everyone has different needs, I have included in this part of the book a number of suggestions for navigating the stress that inevitably comes with planning for that long walk down the wedding aisle. The first set of recommendations for sailing through the process is to approach this whole getting-married business equipped with a few tools, some you hopefully can add to your Bridal Stress Survival Kit:

- **Exercise.** As mentioned throughout this book, physical activity is helpful in relieving stress (ever been to a kickboxing class?), improving your immune system, and getting a good night's sleep. It also can be meditative and can help you feel better about yourself and others.

- **Find a confidante you can trust.** This should be someone who will tell you the truth, not just what you want to hear. You need to keep an open mind and know that not everything this person tells you will be easy to hear.

- **Recognize that there are some things you cannot change.** Accept them for what they are. For example, you just may have to accept that your inconsiderate uncle who tells off-color jokes probably won't change for your wedding.

- **Be prepared to compromise.** Yes, you are the bride and it is your wedding, but you still will need to compromise on some things. Choose your battles carefully, and make sure the battles you choose to fight or let go of are ones that could really make a difference in how you remember your wedding.

- **Look for the good in situations instead of the bad.** See the glass as half full, not as half empty.

- **Learn to say no to yourself and others.** Don't promise too much. Give yourself enough time to get necessary tasks done or delegate them to those you trust (and then let go).

- **Laugh.** Laugh often and try to find the humor in your experiences. Bringing your sense of humor to a tense situation can help you "reframe" the issue and find a new solution.

- **Get plenty of sleep.** Life always looks different when you are rested. Your body needs time to renew itself, especially when it's under tremendous pressure.

- **Set aside time for yourself.** Take a few hours for a walk in a place you love, or get a massage, facial, or manicure. Such activities all feel good and help you rejuvenate.

- **Have fun.** This is the best coping strategy of all. Have fun, enjoy, and create great memories.

Sure, this list sounds great. But perhaps it may not be so easy to remember when your caterer calls to cancel on you two weeks before your wedding day. But that is when you need to remember—and use—the personal coping strategies that you've developed. If you've planned ahead and created a list of tactics you will deploy during those unexpected bumps in the road, you will be ready and able to ride them out. If you keep your Bridal Stress Survival Kit close at hand, you can pull it out at any time you feel your face turning red and your blood pressure rising.

CHAPTER 20

Stress-reduction Exercises

Many of us tend to ignore stress, insisting that we are OK. However, it is imperative to acknowledge when we are stressed. It's very hard to deal with something stressful when we can't admit it exists. Once you have identified that you are stressed, try to find the best way for you to cope with it. You may need more than one favorite tactic. When stressed, I find doing some breathing exercises or soothing stretches to be beneficial. Following are some breathing and stretching exercises that you can select from and use when you need them most.

Breathing Exercises

The following are two breathing exercises to help you relax and de-stress.

Breathing Your Body Away

Sit on the floor with your feet straight in front of you with your toes pointed to the ceiling. Gently focus your attention on your feet and legs. Be aware of all the sensations you feel in your feet and legs. Inhale a long, slow breath, and as you do, breathe in all those sensations. In your mind's eye, imagine that you are erasing this part of your body. Now, as you exhale, breathe out all those sensations. Once again, breathe in your feet and legs, and exhale them from your body so that in your mind, you can see yourself only from your hips up.

Now, with another long breath, breathe in all the parts of your body from your neck down, and as you exhale, breathe them away. Begin with your fingers. Breathe in your fingers, hands, wrists and arms; then exhale them away.

Now move on to your neck and head. As you breathe in, imagine your neck and head being erased, and then exhale to breathe them away.

Finally, return to focusing on your entire body in one breath, beginning with the feet. Take a long, slow breath in, and as you do, erase any little parts of your body that still remain in your mind's eye. Let a long, slow breath out, and as you exhale, breathe away all the remaining parts. Then just sit quietly for a minute and enjoy feeling yourself deeply relaxed.

Rag Doll Breathing Exercise

Stand up, wherever you are. Reach your arms over your head, close your eyes, and inhale through your nose until your lungs are full. Once your lungs are full and you are at a full body stretch, drop forward slowly like a rag doll. Bend your knees slightly, release your tension, exhale, and let your fingers touch the floor, completely relaxed—just like a rag doll. Repeat this breathing exercise one to three more times.

Three Minutes of Stretching You Can Do Anywhere

Here are five stretches you can do in the car, at your desk, on a plane . . . anywhere.

1. Stand or sit, and reach your arms overhead with your fingers extended to the ceiling. Take a deep breath through your nose and exhale through your mouth. Keep shifting your reach from left arm to right arm, extending to the sky or ceiling.

2. Remain standing or seated and interlace your fingers. Hold your arms straight out in front of you at shoulder height. Turn your palms away from you, and drop your head (with eyes closed) so that your chin rests on your

chest. Reach your arms out so that your shoulders get a good stretch across your upper back. You can roll your head from side to side as well if that feels good. Do this while taking long breaths in and out of your nose.

3. Stand with your knees slightly bent or remain seated, and interlace your fingers behind your back. Close your eyes, drop your head back (only as far as comfortable), stick out your chest, and raise your interlaced hands upward as far as is comfortable. Take long breaths, in through your nose and out through your mouth.

4. Sit on a chair, bench, or exercise ball. Keep one foot flat on the floor while extending the other leg out in front of you so that only your heel touches the floor. Drop your chest toward your thigh until you feel a pull in the back of your upper leg (your hamstring), and extend your fingers toward your toes. Hold this position for 30 seconds, breathing in through your nose and out through your mouth. Repeat with your other leg.

5. Still seated, slowly twist your whole body as far around to the right or the left as it will go comfortably. Now slowly twist in the opposite direction. Keep your feet on the floor in front of you while you are twisting. Be careful to twist only to a comfortable point.

Tension-reducing Exercise

Relaxation is the opposite of tension. You can use the following exercise to control tension and enhance relaxation in both your body and your mind.

It will probably be most useful to you if you record the following exercise on tape or digitally and then listen to it, rather than just try to read and remember the various parts of it. If you do choose to record the exercise, be sure to read it slowly, including the pauses indicated in the text, to allow the relaxation to occur.

Use your recording of this exercise only when you are sitting or lying comfortably at home or aren't performing an activity that requires you to be fully alert. Do not use the recoding while driving or operating any kind of machinery.

One of the main activities of this exercise involves alternately tensing and relaxing specific muscle groups. When doing this, be sure you tighten your muscles enough to make them tense but not to cause you pain. Feeling pain means that you are tensing your muscles too much.

Read or listen to the following exercise script while you perform the exercise:

Settle back into a sitting or laying position and get as comfortable as you possibly can. You can be in a chair, on the floor, or on a pillow. Close your eyes gently. Tune in to your breathing. (Pause.) Notice the pace and rhythm of your breath. (Pause.) Take another breath, a little deeper this time, letting yourself feel completely calm, peaceful, comfortable, and relaxed. (Pause.) Now, with the rest of your body feeling more and more comfortable and relaxed, slowly clench your right fist. Clench it tighter and tighter and study the tension. Keep it clenched and feel the tension in your fist, hand, and forearm. (Short pause.) Let your hands relax and go limp, allowing your fingers to become loose. Notice the contrast between the earlier feeling of tension and the present feeling of relaxation. (Short pause.) Let your whole body go and relax even more completely. (Short pause.) Bend both your elbows and tense your biceps. Tense them hard until they almost quiver. Hold them tight and study the tension. (Short pause.) Now straighten out your arms and drop them gently to your sides. Go limp, feeling heavy and relaxed. Notice the tension leave your muscles and experience the relaxation that replaces the tension. Let the feeling flow and spread into the rest of your body so that you feel peaceful and calm. Feel yourself becoming more and more relaxed. (Pause, and from this point onward, pause where it seems appropriate to allow enough time for the tensing and relaxing to occur.)

Focus all your attention on your neck, your shoulders, and your upper back. As you breathe, imagine that you are releasing tension from your neck, shoulders, and upper back. With each breath you take, feel your neck, shoulders, and upper back grow heavier and more and more relaxed. As you release tension in your arms, neck, shoulders, and upper back, feel the wave of relaxation moving downward through your torso, lower back, and stomach. With each breath, you become more and more relaxed.

Now tighten and flex the muscles in your buttocks and thighs. You can flex your thighs by pressing down on your heels with your toes in the air. Hold the tension. Keep the muscles tight and tense. Now let go. Relax and notice the difference as your hips and thighs loosen up, and allow that feeling to progress until you feel completely and deeply relaxed.

Point your toes straight out, away from your body as though you were on tiptoes. Feel the muscles in your calves become taut and tense. Hold the tension. Study the tension. Now relax. Feel the difference between the tension and the delightful, calm, peaceful feeling of being deeply relaxed. Feel the heaviness of your entire lower body as you relax further still.

Relax even more deeply by taking a deep breath and slowly exhaling. As you breathe deeply, feel your entire body become heavy, comfortable, and relaxed. Think the following thoughts to yourself: "I feel quiet. I am feeling deeply relaxed. My body feels calm and quiet. My neck, my jaw, and my forehead are all calm and smooth. My whole body is heavy, comfortable, relaxed, and quiet. My arms and hands are heavy and warm. I am at peace." (At this point, give yourself a few more minutes of deep relaxation before ending the relaxation session.)

After ending the experience, take a deep breath, wiggle your toes, and open your eyes. When you do so, you will feel refreshed and calm.

Other Relaxation Exercises

Here are two more relaxation exercises just for variety.

Smile Exercise

This is my favorite relaxation exercise. You can do it anywhere and it really does make you feel better. You can do it while walking, sitting in class, taking a test, and so on. First, smile. Yes, smile, to remind yourself that you don't actually have all the cares of the world on your shoulders. Then, take a long, deep breath, and let it out slowly. Now take a second long, deep breath, and as you let it out, feel yourself releasing the tensions in your mind and in your body. Just let yourself relax more and more as you continue whatever activity you were doing.

Your Favorite Scene, Place, or Person

Sit comfortably and quietly in a place that allows you to focus internally without interruption. As you're sitting quietly, think of the most relaxing image you can. Perhaps it's a favorite place (a vacation spot or retreat of some sort), or maybe it's a person with whom you feel at peace, or maybe it's a scene (such as a meadow, beach, or mountain retreat)—whatever works for you. Take a few seconds to determine this.

Now see that image or place in your mind. Be sure to notice the good feelings you have when you are in that place or enjoying that image. Let them take over your whole awareness. If your thoughts wander, gently direct them back to that peaceful, relaxing place or image. Breathe slowly and keep your focus on the relaxing scene in your mind. When you are ready, open your eyes, take one more deep breath, and resume your day.

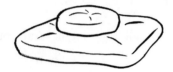

CHAPTER 21

Dealing with the Stress of Planning

~~~~~~

While writing this book, I asked a number of new brides what worked best for them in handling stress during the wedding-planning stages. I've collected some of their best tips in the pages that follow.

Stress Busting Tips from Recent Brides

From Jennifer W, married October 2004:

- Create a website with all the details and info about your wedding so that guests can refer to it instead of bothering you.

- Take time out for you and pamper yourself. I had facials every month for the three months before the wedding. I received relaxation, alone time, and great skin all in one sitting.

- Lean on your attendants, friends, and family and ask for their help. They *want* to help you, even if it's with the little things, like copying off your programs or tying all those bows. Don't be afraid to ask for help or delegate. You cannot get it all done by yourself, and if you try, you won't have any fun.

• Stay organized. Carry a notebook with you that you can write everything in and keep all your information, samples, invoices, etc., in one place. On your laptop or home computer, checklists in Excel also help with keeping things tidy.

• Make time for exercise. You have to, even if you aren't trying to lose weight before your wedding. It's just good for you to help fight stress and keep yourself healthy during such a busy time.

• Above all, remember what this is all about. You are getting *married*. This is about you and your soon-to-be-husband's commitment. The programs, DJ, cake, and gifts are all fun, but they are not what matters the most. Choose your battles and prepare yourself that some things may not go perfectly and you'll just have to let it go. But as long as you and your honey share your vows that day, then you have accomplished the most important part of the day.

From Jennifer B, married September 2004:

• When the wedding planning gets to be too much . . . *go shopping!* I went shopping for the honeymoon as my stress reliever, and the mere act of trying on lingerie and bathing suits helped me to stick to my fitness routine.

From Catherine, married July 2004:

- Be organized: Get a notebook (or a group of folders) and divide it into sections like food, music, printed materials, etc. Clip pictures to put in the folders during planning. That way you will have visuals to show people what you are looking for.

- Keep track of your presents on your computer and immediately send thank-you notes out. . . . Having them build up is stressful.

- Have the type of wedding you and your fiancé want. In the end, that is all that matters. My family wanted us to have a huge formal wedding, and we ended up with an island wedding with 40 people . . . it was perfect and our families loved it.

- Get a dress you want and that you are comfortable in. I bought a dress with my mom and sister that I thought I liked, but every time I tried it on it just did not feel like me. I ended up getting a simple sheath that I loved and stressed about telling my parents. They just laughed when I told them, so I stressed about it for months and they did not care.

- Hire a wedding planner. We hired someone to handle the day-of details. The best thing I ever did . . . I woke up on the day of my wedding not worried about a thing.

- Don't let your wedding plans consume you. Work out, eat right, continue to do the things you love. It is easy to get overwhelmed with it all.

- Focus on what is important to you—for us that was a good venue, music, and food. The rest we compromised on due to budget, such as flowers. (We had a local flower grower do the flowers, which saved us money.) All the little details seem like a big deal, but your guests will not notice.

- With everything you do, they will notice if the bride and groom are relaxed and having fun.

- Engage your fiancé and don't be a control freak. My fiancé was *very* opinionated, which totally stressed me out. In the end I just learned to not be a control freak and let him plan the things he wanted to, like the food. It was probably the most stressful thing for me but in the end it was just fine.

What About Mom?

Here are some words of wisdom from mothers of the bride.

- Don't take every suggestion, comment, or remark personally. Let all the extra information roll off your back, and consider how much you have looked forward to planning this.

- Don't start a crash diet in hopes of fitting into the "small" dress you want. Your husband will enjoy you much more if you are relaxed and healthy than if you are stressed and too skinny to hold yourself up at the altar.

- Keep with your daily routine of healthy eating, exercise, and keeping calm.

- Remember to take time for yourself and your mom— you are in this together. Remember, she has been dreaming of this day since she found out she was having a girl.

- Delegate—and trust those you delegate to. You must remember, the more you try to do on your own, the more you will stress.

- Keep the word "humor" in your vocabulary. If you lose that sense of humor, wonderful laugh, beautiful smile, and calm attitude, people will not want to be around you or do things for you.

- Remember this day is not just about your husband-to-be, his family, or your family and friends; it is also about *you*. It is not a life-threatening experience, just the beginning of the life experience you have dreamed of.

- Exercise daily, walk in the fresh air, start the day with a prayer, and take a deep breath before heading off to work.

- Get lots of rest, not just dog-tired sleep, but healthy rest. Take small breaks throughout the day, and go into a room alone and think of all the excitement you will have when the Big Day arrives. Organize your schedule to include downtime for yourself.

- Relax, refresh, renew. Relax the body, refresh the mind, renew the spirit, and take a tea break. Love, love, love, and more love!

Tips from the Field

Following are top tips for brides from experts in the field you will most likely be dealing with: dress consultants, photographers, florists, caterers, and wedding planners. Not surprisingly, many of them offered the same advice. I included the redundancy of their statements because it really drives home these points and gives you a better idea of what to do—and what not to do.

From dress consultants, on choosing your dress:

- The first time you go to shop for your dress, bring a small group or go alone. This will allow you to make some decisions for yourself without a flurry of other opinions influencing you.

- Try on all the styles so that you can see for yourself which dress type looks the best on you.

- Keep an open mind. Don't get stuck on one dress that you saw in a magazine. It might not flatter you. Most brides come in with a specific dress in mind and leave with something different.

- Keep your top two to five dresses in the running and let the others drop off. It's too hard to manage a top 10 list.

- Narrow down your decision to a few dresses and then bring in your mom, bridesmaids, and others for the final vote.

- Don't buy into the myth that it will be "love at first sight" with your dress; this does not actually happen very often.

- Remember to choose a dress according to how it makes you feel before anything else. If it feels great, you will look great.

- Have fun when you are trying on wedding dresses. This should be a fun activity—enjoy it.

- Make sure your shoes are as comfortable as possible. You will be in them a long time, and they are not "on stage" as much as you might think.

- Always ask for a discount. The dress consultant has more flexibility than you think. Especially ask if you are buying your dress and your bridesmaid's dresses from the same vendor.

From dress consultants, on choosing bridesmaid dresses:

- Don't worry too much about this. It is your day, and you can add straps to any dress so all of your bridesmaids feel comfortable.

- Have at least two of your bridesmaids vote on the dress they will wear.

- Some brides are now just giving a color and a fabric type and then allowing the bridesmaids to choose their own style.

From photographers:

- Make sure you choose a photographer with whom you feel comfortable. You should "connect" with your photographer and feel that he or she sees the same vision you do.

- Do a lot of preparation. Then let go and allow your photographer to do his or her job. If you have done the work up front, the day-of should go well, and you can feel confident that everything will turn out just as you hoped it would.

- Make a list of your must-have photos. Keep the list succinct and prioritize it for your photographer. This way you will get the shots you want the most, and you set your photographer up for success in meeting your needs.

- Surround yourself with people who are supportive and practical so that if something does go wrong, you have others who can run interference for you and you can continue to enjoy the day.

- Assign an assertive friend or family member to be your photographer's assistant. This person can help make decisions and knows what is important to you.

- If something goes wrong, just keep going and try to laugh, laugh, laugh . . . it makes for great photos!

From florists:

- Be organized and give yourself plenty of time and space to get the job done. You can book your florist far, far in advance and work on the specific details nearer to your wedding date.

- Hire the best person you can find who has experience and can foresee problems before they arise. Maybe Aunt Jean makes magic in the garden, but that does not always translate into setting up the floral arrangements for an entire wedding.

- Trust your florist. He or she has experience and truly wants to do a great job for you. Your florist will let you know what he or she needs to meet and exceed your expectations. Trust your florist to do the job you have hired him or her to do.

- Arrive at the meeting with your florist with ideas, but be flexible. Your florist has experience with lots of weddings and may have ideas for you that will work better for your specific venue, season, or timeline.

- Remember that you are planning a marriage, and the flowers (and everything else) are really secondary. If you are happy, relaxed, and enjoying yourself, everything else will look great to your guests.

From caterers:

- People who know "exactly what they want" tend to be more stressed out. Keep an open mind.

- Hire a good catering company, and let them do what they do best.

- Keep things simple; this tends to lead to a more successful event.

- Keep your expectations in line with your budget.

- Don't micromanage. Communicate your vision, and then let go.

- If you delegate oversight of the caterer to someone else you trust, step out of the process and let that person be the contact for the caterer.

- Communicate your expectations and timeline clearly and up front.

- Choose a caterer who loves to do weddings. He or she will do the best job for you.

- Explore all the things the caterer can line up for you—rentals, linens, and so on—so that you or someone else does not have to worry about these items.

- Remember, the food is only a small part of the day and should not be a make-or-break part of it.

From wedding planners:

The wedding planners I talked to had similar recommendations for brides. Here is a top 10 list of their best advice.

1. **Prioritize.** Not everything is the number-one priority for your wedding memories. Make sure you focus on the most important items first.

2. **Set a realistic budget.** This will help eliminate a lot of stress for you and avoid misunderstandings with the professionals you hire to help with your wedding. Happy vendors make for a happy event.

3. **Plan ahead and communicate, communicate, communicate.** If you must have Vendela roses and not just white, don't assume your florist knows it. Be prepared to offer a thoughtful rationale for your plans as you review them with your families, and be open to their ideas.

4. **Remember that your friends and family are there for *you*.** They're not there for the cake, the party favors, or the dinner.

5. **Be organized.** Try to find a way to be organized, even if you are not an organized person.

6. **Remember, it's not just *your* day.** It's also your groom's, your mom's, his mom's, your friends', and that of everyone who cares about you.

7. **Find a great team of wedding professionals.** These people have great insight and lots of experience regarding what really happens on the Big Day and what generally works best. Don't be afraid to ask them to find creative ways to accomplish what you'd like.

8. **Laugh a lot.** Enjoy the process.

9. **Take care of yourself.** A tired, unhealthy bride is a stressed bride.

10. **Remember to eat on your wedding day.** It will help you stay energized and feeling good.

Other Ways to De-stress

All the sage advice from recent brides, their moms, and experts in the field can only help. But even if you follow their advice to the letter, stress will still seep in. Here are some other ideas for ways you can cope with the pressure. Feel free to put any of these in your Stress Survival Kit.

- **Do yoga.** This is a favorite stress-reducing activity for many people in the world. Join a class that is convenient for you and enjoyable. If you don't have time for a class, try a home video or DVD. (This is the easiest way for me to enjoy yoga.) Many yoga videos and DVDs are very good, and the ease of doing your workout at home can be a great stress reducer in itself. My personal favorite yoga instructor on DVD is Rodney Yee.

- **Get a massage.** Having someone work on your body for an hour or more is a great indulgence. A massage therapist can help work out knots and release points of tension in your body that you did not even know were there. As with a doctor, ask for recommendations from friends and family. Finding a good masseuse is key to making this hour or more worthwhile.

- **Have a facial, manicure, or pedicure.** These small moments of renewal do not cost a lot of money. Plus, they feel good and make you feel renewed, refreshed, and pretty.

- **Spend a few moments of each day in quiet meditation.** There are numerous books, tapes, and websites that can teach you how to meditate. Taking this time away from your normal (and perhaps hectic) life can help reduce stress and anxiety and can help improve your immune system.

- **Keep a journal.** Another way many people deal with stress is by journaling. Writing in a journal gives you a way to release your thoughts and experiences. Many find this fulfilling and cathartic. Many books, tapes, and websites can help you learn how to most effectively journal your stress away.

CHAPTER 22

Stress and the Healthy Bride Program

W
e started this book with a chapter on change management. We discussed the stages of change and how to move from a sedentary to an active lifestyle. If you are still reading this book and are following the program I have outlined in it, you may want to look at what types of stress you are experiencing from undergoing all this change.

Change is not easy for human beings. We seem to really love and need routine. If the last time you exercised was in eighth-grade gym class and you're now in your twenties or thirties and are getting ready for a wedding, you have a lot of time of inactivity to redirect. Be nice to yourself and give yourself the time to develop a new set of routines. As you already know, this will not happen naturally. Instead, you'll need to apply some energy toward making these changes work for you. This change process of moving from a less healthy to a healthier lifestyle will also involve a bit of stress.

A large part of success in weight loss seems to hinge on your internal voice and how it speaks to you during times of anxiety and stress. Being positive is a huge part of success in weight loss. Developing ways to deal with the stresses of life can help you stay on track. In this part of the book, you read the words of wisdom from past brides who have had success in staying happy and on track during their wedding-planning process. And by now, you have created and are carrying your Stress Survival Kit with you, which means you have some great diversions and exercises you can deploy when stress sneaks up on you.

Many of the recommendations for managing stress are very basic, such as eating a healthy diet, getting enough rest, and maintaining a regular exercise program. The hard part is listening to yourself and checking your stress level (by using the test from the beginning of this chapter); turning to your friends, family, and fiancé for advice and assistance; and not allowing yourself to get run down, burned out, or harried. You want to be happy and relaxed on your wedding day—make this a fun process and enjoy the journey.

Many of the wedding experts I interviewed for the book recalled the one bride who was their worst nightmare. They described her as a controlling, do-it-all-herself, overly involved Bridezilla who drove herself crazy and in the end couldn't wait for her wedding day to be over. Yikes! You can avoid being this person, especially now that you have so many ideas and suggestions for ways to reduce stress and cope with the pressure of planning your wedding (and building your marriage). The Bridal Stress Survival Kit you've created for yourself will help guide you to peace, happiness, health, and a blissful journey to the altar and beyond.

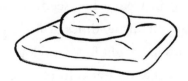

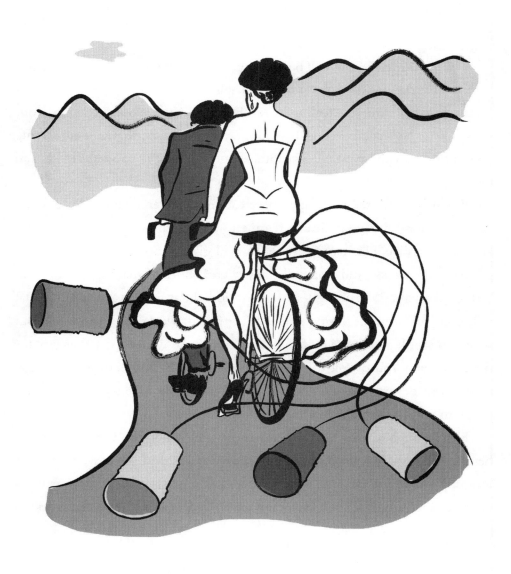

When you started the Healthy Bride pro-gram, you stated your fitness vows out loud and you committed to them.

The trick now will be remembering what you said and sticking to the promises you made yourself.

Are you feeling as motivated today as you did before your walk down the wedding aisle? If so, hooray! It's fantastic that you are staying committed to your vows and keeping your "marriage" to your fitness and health intact.

If you are less fired up, don't worry too much. Even feeling a little moti-vated to stick with your health regimen after reaching your wedding-day goal is impressive. This part of the book will give you that push you need to get back on track—and hopefully stay there. Short of marriage, your 40th birthday, or your 25-year high-school reunion, there are few things in life that will keep you from declining that third or fourth workout of the week. But when you look fabulous, you feel fabulous, and you want to stay that way for the long term. You owe it to yourself to take care of number one every day for the rest of your life. The commitment you made when you started this program was to yourself, and my dear, you deserve it.

First, though, the bad news: Now is the time when the hard work really begins. Admit it, it was pretty easy to stay on track with your wedding date looming and everything in your life focused on making you and your wed-ding celebration look, feel, and smell good. You have come so far, working hard to get yourself into good physical, mental, and nutritional shape. And now, I want to give you the tools to help you stay there.

You may be wondering how you will stay motivated without that looming Big Day goal. Happily, this section of the book provides tips and tools that can help prevent you from backsliding.

The Honeymoon and Beyond

Perhaps you are reading this chapter before jetting off to your exotic honeymoon destination. Perhaps you feel a bit nervous, knowing you'll either be wearing a bathing suit or showing plenty of skin during this vacation of a lifetime. But you shouldn't worry. If you have followed the Healthy Bride program, you have developed great workout habits. And they have served you well—you look and feel great!

If you're feeling really motivated, there's no reason you cannot take your workout with you. On your honeymoon, you'll have all the time in the world to do whatever you want. If you're still preparing or packing for the trip, bring your workout band with you if you think you may use it. (You can also use the travel workout exercises supplied in Appendix C.) I understand this may be asking a lot . . . after all, you are on your honeymoon! So if you want to take a break from your resistance band and dumbbells, by all means do.

Instead of doing specific workouts on your honeymoon, you can get the exercise you need just by walking. When you travel, you usually end up walking a ton anyway and that certainly counts as exercise. If you are going somewhere sunny and near water, you are probably swimming, perhaps every day—this also counts. Go hiking, or rent bikes, canoes, or kayaks. Don't worry too much about working out per se—just build fun activities into each day, and you'll find yourself getting natural cardio workouts without even having to plan them. These are all activities you and your new husband can enjoy together.

It's easy to work in enough exercise while on the road. You just have to be committed to staying active. Eating well is the same story. You can eat well *and* enjoy your meals while on the road—and on your honeymoon. Have anything you want; just remember to enjoy food and alcohol in moderation. You may also want to review the Dining Out: Tips to Guide You through the Menu section on page 136 before you leave for your trip.

Return from the Honeymoon

After the honeymoon ends, life will eventually return to the old routine. Make sure you are thinking about the new, healthy you when you get back home. You will to need to talk to yourself in the voice of the healthy person who exercises, eats well, and takes care of herself. Remember, you want to remain this person. You don't want to slide back to the stage in your life where you were always thinking of being more healthy but never doing anything about it. (Remember the Precontemplative stage?)

A number of brides I've worked with before their weddings lost some of that prenuptial momentum for exercising after their weddings were over. Their focus on staying healthy and feeling good seemed to have drifted off. But if you were able to fit in exercise and good meals before your wedding, you can certainly do it after the wedding, too. You just need a new goal to get you moving.

What you need to do right away is to take an inventory. Revisit the Physical Activity Stages of Change Questionnaire on page 5 to see where you are now, and use this information to set new goals. Don't wait.

This is also a good time to review your lifetime fitness goals. These may help you stay on track for the long term. It's hard to think ahead to being an elderly person, but what you do now really does affect your later years. For example, one of my own lifetime goals is to still be hiking the trails of the Pacific Northwest when I am in my seventies. One of yours may be, "I want to stay fit enough so that I can play soccer with my children." These are only ideas; your lifestyle and personal situation will dictate what your personal long-term goals are today, and they will probably change as you get older.

After the honeymoon and upon returning to everyday life, you will have the greatest temptation to fall back into the not-so-healthy lifestyle you had before picking up this book. Because I don't want that to happen, I have provided in this part of the book some tactics you can use to stay on track after the honeymoon is over.

Setting New Goals and Avoiding a Backslide

You know how to set good goals, and you have practiced and been successful at achieving them. The challenge at this point will be staying committed to those goals. I suggest creating another looming deadline for yourself. Sure, it will not be a deadline quite as looming as your wedding date, but you can try to create other deadlines that will give you the nudge, nudge, push, push you need to get back into the routine of taking good care of yourself. Make it a big goal, such as signing up for a 5K race, a mini-triathlon, the ski bus, a tennis tournament, a hiking vacation, or whatever it is that will get you excited and keep you on your exercise and healthy eating program. By putting yourself in a situation where turning back can have repercussions (remember saying "yes" to your fiancé?), you will be more likely to stay on track.

If it will help, get your best friend to join you in your endeavor (though make sure she wants to do this and is committed to the goal). She can help you get and stay on track.

This goal will feel different from your wedding-day goal because when you achieve it you may be part of a crowd of people with similar goals; you're not the focal point anymore, unlike when you were when you were the bride on your wedding day. You will not have the same amount of pressure, and to be perfectly honest, you can decide to give up on your goal without anyone noticing . . . except for you, that is. To avoid losing motivation, it is helpful to tell everyone you know what your goal is. They will ask you how you are coming along with your goal and will be cheering for you along the way.

Keep up the commitment you have made to be a healthy person. Don't forget how good it feels to set and achieve goals. Yes, it's work, but isn't it less work than it was when you first started this program?

How to Handle a Backslide

What if you find yourself slipping backward? How will you notice? Pay attention to your inner voice. Is it saying, "Let's go"? Or is the voice inside your head saying, "I can't, won't, don't feel like it . . . " or "I knew I wouldn't . . . "? If you fail to uphold your vows, you are going to feel terrible. It will reduce your self-esteem, your self-image, and your coping skills. Plus, your inner voice will start dragging you down instead of propping you up.

Don't get too upset if you have a couple of days or weeks where you lose focus. This is OK as long as you look inward and figure out what is happening. There are times in life where other commitments and events can get in the way. The first thing you need to do is to figure out whether you are in a backslide or just having a temporary motivation problem. A backslide lasts longer than a few days, and you will probably know when you are in one. You are not eating healthy foods, you are not exercising, and your old, bad habits are starting to replace your new healthy habits.

Now is the time to go find that Buck the Backslide Kit you began to create early on in the book on page 9, when you were feeling terrifically motivated. Use this kit now to help you get back into a positive mindset. Start by reading through the goals and statements you wrote down. This should give you enough inspiration to kick yourself back into gear. If not, there may be some strong obstacles to exercise at work in your life right now. The next section will help you examine some of these scenarios.

Some Reasons You May Be in a Backslide

The following are some of the most common reasons you may be in a backslide:

- You are sick.

- You have been recently been injured.

- You recently experienced a family emergency.

- You are having difficulty coping with the issues in your life right now.

- You are having trouble managing your eating (and drinking) behavior in public, at parties, or elsewhere.

Being sick or injured are perfectly good reasons to take some time away from your exercise program. However, in most cases, you should still be able to continue with your healthy eating program. Taking care of your body in every way is most important. Once you are feeling better or are fully healed, return to your exercise program as soon as possible to stop the backslide from snowballing.

A family emergency also may put strain on your regular exercise schedule for a while, but it is also a time when you must be careful to take very good care of yourself. The stresses you endure during these times of crises are immense, and exercise and healthy eating are more important than ever to get you through.

Be sure to keep your Bridal Stress Survival Kit easily accessible. Though you created it to get you through the planning of your wedding, this kit can help you during all times of stress and emotional upheaval. Keep it relevant, updated, and useful for you. Revisit the stress management section of the book any time you need new ideas for relaxation techniques.

A final word: Managing your behavior at parties, events, vacations, and holidays may take practice. If you have too much to eat or drink at a particular event, don't throw in the towel and start saying you are through with your health program. You need to take charge of your inner voice and get it talking to you in a way that motivates you to be the healthy person you want. A small setback is not a crisis; it's just a setback. Forget about the extra piece of fudge you ate and keep forging ahead. In the end, one transgression will not matter.

Reframing Your Inner Voice

Perhaps the most common reason for backsliding is that your motivation and desire for fitness and good health have waned, and you're being plagued by an inner voice that makes excuses for you not exercising. That voice in your head has some serious power. For this reason, it is key that you find a way to respond to this voice, so you can get yourself back on track. The trick is to listen to what your inner voice is saying and then "reframe" it.

For example, let's say that you set a goal to work out three times a week. This is less often than you were working out before your wedding, but life post-honeymoon is still a little crazy and you are giving yourself a little time to work back up to your five workouts per week. The problem you are having is that after two workouts, your inner voice is battling with you over making the third trip to the treadmill. Here is a list of some possible excuses your inner voice may be making, with a reframed (more positive, motivating) version of each.

Inner voice: I don't want to go to the gym. I am tired and I don't feel like working out.

Reframe: I am tired right now, but by going to the gym I will feel energized and will feel really good about working out three times this week.

Inner voice: I hate that dumb treadmill. I am getting so bored just running on that thing.

Reframe: I am getting tired of working on the treadmill, so I am going to do only 10 minutes on it and then do 10 minutes each on three additional machines I am not as used to. This will give me a different workout for my body and my mind today.

Inner voice: I would really like to just sit on the couch and watch Oprah.

Reframe: I can go to the gym, bring my headphones, and watch Oprah while I am working out. In fact, from now on, I will only watch Oprah when working out so that I will look forward to my workouts!

You get the idea. It is possible to reframe your internal voice so that you are being kind and encouraging to yourself. Be aware of that internal voice and make sure it is lifting you up, not dragging you down.

Balancing Shoulds and Wants

Another problem you may be facing is that you are truly having a hard time fitting exercise and healthy eating into your hectic schedule. If so, it may be time to look at the balance in your life between *wants* and *shoulds*. Wants are the things we desire to do, such as exercise, garden, paint—really anything that gives you joy. Shoulds are things we must do, such as grocery shop, work, do laundry, and pay bills. Your goal should be to balance the two categories so that the number of wants in your life is equal to the number of shoulds.

To do this, make a list of all the things you do in a given day. Put all the wants in one column and all the shoulds in another column. What do your lists look like? Are they equal?

You need to direct enough energy inward (toward your wants) so that your life includes personal pleasure, satisfaction, and fulfillment. You are a new bride and you are establishing a new life. Now is the time to make sure you are getting what you need.

If your shoulds list is longer than your wants list, you have some work to do. If you can't think of any activities you love to do, this is a red flag—you really need to do some checking in with yourself to make sure you are nurturing and taking care of number one. You *do* have a choice. You might not think so, but you do. It may mean asking for help from others, adjusting your schedule, or getting more assistance from your spouse. Do whatever it takes to get your life in balance.

Brainstorming New Goals

Perhaps you may be having difficulty coming up with new goals by which to gauge your health and fitness program and motivate yourself. This final section suggests some possible goals you may want to aim for.

Do you want to be able to run three miles without stopping? Run a 5K or a marathon? How about completing a walk for an organization that you feel passionate about?

There are many wonderful websites full of ideas for physical adventures you can train for and use to blow away the limitations you thought you had. Here are just a few of the sites:

- www.active.com
- www.arthritis.org/events/jointsinmotion/default.asp
- www.balancebaradventure.com
- www.bikelane.com
- www.bikewalk.org
- www.care2.com
- www.hiketohealth.com
- www.womenclimbing.com/climb/events.asp

Your goal, though, doesn't have to be event-oriented. Maybe your goal is to be able to play tag with your children or grandchildren or to keep up with your husband on a mountain bike ride. Whatever the goal, keep on going, and keep setting and resetting goals that make sense for your life. And at all times, keep those wants balanced with the many shoulds life brings.

Use the following text to set your next goal. Go ahead and write it down on a separate piece of paper.

> My goal is to (do) _____ by (date) _____.
> I will get to that goal by following the program I designed using my own workout schedule for the next six weeks. In six weeks, I will evaluate my progress, make changes, and continue moving toward my end date.

As you continue to live your new healthy life, remember that it's OK to take good care of yourself—just for you. You deserve the best, every single day, from this day forward.

Appendix A

Recommended Serving Sizes and Balanced Food Pyramid

Use the following lists and balanced food pyramid as guidelines to meeting your nutritional needs. Each food group is shown with the number of servings to aim for each day. The food group lists also contain a sampling of serving sizes of particular foods or dishes so that you can see what counts as one serving. Use these lists to determine your portion sizes and the number servings you should have in one day. The key is to have a variety of foods from the different food groups to get the widest range of nutrients.

Whole Grains

Goal: 6-11 servings per day

One serving equals any of the following:

- 1 slice of whole-grain bread
- 1 corn tortilla or whole-wheat tortilla
- ½ whole-grain bagel, English muffin, or bun
- ½ whole-wheat pita pocket
- ½ cup cooked grain (brown rice, barley, quinoa, or millet)
- ½ cup cooked whole-wheat pasta, brown-rice pasta, or quinoa
- 1 cup ready-to-eat breakfast cereal
- ½ cup cooked breakfast cereal (oats, amaranth, or millet)

Vegetables

Goal: 3-5 servings per day or unlimited amount of leafy greens and other nonstarchy vegetables

One serving equals any of the following:

- 1 cup raw vegetables (romaine, red- and green-leaf lettuce, spinach, or cabbage)
- ½ cup cooked vegetables (broccoli, leafy greens, or cabbage)
- ¾ cup vegetable juice (low-sodium preferred)
- ¾ cup starchy vegetables (potatoes, peas, corn, sweet potatoes, or yams) in moderation (2 servings or less per day)

Fruits

Goal: 2-4 servings per day

One serving equals any of the following:

- 1 apple, medium (2¾ in. diameter)
- 1 pear, medium (6½ oz)
- 1 banana, medium (7-8 in. long)
- 1 orange, medium (3 in. diameter)
- ½ cup berries
- 15 grapes
- ½ grapefruit, medium (4 in. diameter)
- ½ cup chopped fruit

Protein

Goal: 2-3 servings per day

One serving equals any of the following:
- 2-3 oz of cooked fish, poultry, or meat
- ½ cup cooked dried beans (includes lentils and peas)
- 3-4 oz tofu
- 2 tablespoons nut butter (peanut, almond, cashew, or sesame tahini)
- 1 large egg
- ⅓ cup nuts

Calcium Sources

Goal: 1,000–1,200 mg of calcium per day

- 1 cup cooked dark leafy greens (collards, kale, chard, or spinach) = 100–200 mg calcium
- 1 cup cooked broccoli = 90 mg calcium
- 3-4 oz tofu = 200–600 mg calcium (check the ingredient list for calcium sulfate or calcium chloride, these will have calcium)
- 2 tablespoons almond butter = 90 mg calcium
- 1 oz or 24 almonds= 72 mg calcium
- 1 cup calcium-enriched soymilk or rice milk = 300 mg calcium
- 1 cup nonfat or low-fat yogurt = 250–450 mg calcium
- 1 oz cheese = 150–220 mg calcium
- 1 cup nonfat milk = 300 mg calcium

Note: Some find it difficult to meet this amount of calcium by food alone. In this case, add calcium with vitamin D supplement to meet your needs.

Water

Goal: 8–12 cups per day (may be increased with fluid losses from exercise)

Fat Intake

Goals:

- Less than 20–35% of total calories from fat
- Less than 10% of total calories from saturated fat

Balanced Food Pyramid

If you are more visually inclined, the Balanced Food Pyramid also shows the number of servings in each food group to aim for each day. You may find it helpful to copy this and place on your refrigerator as a daily reminder. Refer to the recommended serving sizes for details about each food group.

The food pyramid shown here is loosely based on the "Healthy Eating Pyramid" from *Eat, Drink, and Be Healthy*, by Walter C. Willett, MD, copyright Simon & Schuster, 2001. That pyramid was created by nutrition experts from the Harvard School of Public Health (HSPH) and should not be confused with the original Food Guide Pyramid created by the USDA. In 2005, the USDA retired this somewhat flawed pyramid, and introduced MyPyramid, a Web-based program that requires consumers to visit the MyPyramid.gov website to receive individualized details for a balanced diet. Though there is much merit in MyPyramid, there are also some noticeable flaws, which are wonderfully detailed on HSPH's website www.hsph.harvard.edu/nutrition source/pyramids.html. As such, we have chosen a modified version of HSPH's "Healthy Eating Pyramid," which offers a much stronger and informative "at-a-glance" representation of a balanced diet. Our modifications to that pyramid illustrate the whole foods-based nutrition program in our book. It emphasizes whole grains, lean protein sources from both meat and non-meat sources, dairy and non-dairy sources of calcium (for those who are lactose intolerant or have dairy intolerances), and high-quality fruits and vegetables.

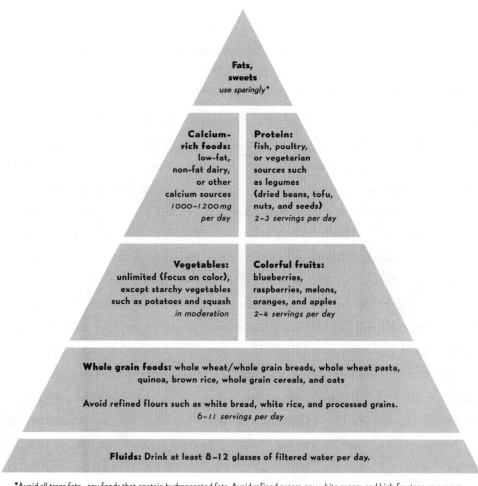

Fats, sweets
*use sparingly**

Calcium-rich foods: low-fat, non-fat dairy, or other calcium sources *1000–1200mg per day*

Protein: fish, poultry, or vegetarian sources such as legumes (dried beans, tofu, nuts, and seeds) *2–3 servings per day*

Vegetables: unlimited (focus on color), except starchy vegetables such as potatoes and squash *in moderation*

Colorful fruits: blueberries, raspberries, melons, oranges, and apples *2–4 servings per day*

Whole grain foods: whole wheat/whole grain breads, whole wheat pasta, quinoa, brown rice, whole grain cereals, and oats

Avoid refined flours such as white bread, white rice, and processed grains. *6–11 servings per day*

Fluids: Drink at least 8–12 glasses of filtered water per day.

*Avoid all trans fats—any foods that contain hydrogenated fats. Avoid refined sugars, any white sugars, and high-fructose corn syrup.

Appendix B

Healthy Bride Recipes

Here are some quick and easy recipes to try. They provide a nice introduction to preparing foods with healthy fats, whole grains, fruit, and vegetables. As you gain experience with these recipes, I encourage you to modify them and create new recipes to your own taste.

Note: It can sometimes be difficult to locate whole foods ingredients like the ones in the following recipes. Some may be found in the local grocery store; if they are not in the general aisles they may be found in bulk foods or the natural foods section, if your store has these. You may ask your local grocer to stock these whole foods ingredients if they currently don't carry these items. Other options are to check the health or natural foods stores in your area, or to use the Internet to search for mail-order sites that sell the ingredients.

Energizing Fruit Smoothie

Use this smoothie as a way to increase your fiber and fruit intake. I like this smoothie as a pre-exercise snack to energize me through my workout program without making me feel overly full. It serves as a great afternoon energy-boosting snack, too. This is a single-serving smoothie recipe, so you won't be tempted to overindulge. Use a banana with other fruit to give this smoothie the right sweetness and creaminess.

¾ cup milk (nonfat milk, soymilk, or rice milk)

½ cup fruit (your choice of berries, pineapple, oranges, or a
   combination of these)

½ medium banana

⅓ cup nonfat plain yogurt

Ice (optional)

Tip: When fruit is not as abundant or in season, frozen fruit can be used. A wide variety of frozen berries is usually available at your grocery store. Put all ingredients into a blender and blend on high until smooth. Serve immediately.

Optional additions:

1 tablespoon wheat germ (contains fiber and added
   nutrients)
1 tablespoon ground raw flaxseeds (contains fiber and
omega-3 fatty acids)
1 teaspoon flaxseed oil (contains omega-3 fatty acids)
1 teaspoon blackstrap molasses (contains sweetener and iron)

Preparation time: 10 minutes

Servings: 1

Nutritional analysis (per serving with nonfat milk and no optional ingredients): Calories, 230; fat, 1 g; cholesterol, 10 mg; sodium, 160 mg; carbohydrates, 45 g; sugar, 37 g; fiber, 3 g; protein, 12 g; calcium, 400 mg

Oat and Millet Hot Cereal with Fruit

This hot cereal is a good introduction to cooking with whole grains. Whole grains are higher in amino acids and fiber. Combining these whole grains with oats (steel-cut or rolled) makes for a creamy cereal. This recipe uses millet, which can be replaced with your choice of whole grain. Millet is an easy grain to digest; it also is a good source of magnesium and B vitamins. The longer it cooks, the creamier it gets. This recipe can be cooked in advance and stored in the refrigerator to be reheated for a quick breakfast.

½ cup millet

½ cup steel-cut oats

3½ cups water

Dash of sea salt

Additional water or milk, as needed

1 small apple or pear, cored and chopped

Maple syrup or honey, to taste

Using a fine strainer, rinse millet under cool water. Put millet and oats into a medium sauce pan with water and salt. Bring to a boil. Reduce heat to a simmer (water will be bubbling slightly). Stir occasionally to prevent grains from sticking to bottom of pot. Cover and cook for 45 to 60 minutes; add more water if mixture gets too thick. Add apple during the last 10 minutes of cooking time. Add sweetener and serve hot.

Tip: Store leftovers in a covered container in the refrigerator, and reheat to serve. Add more liquid as needed for a quick breakfast. Will keep for up to 4 days.

Serving suggestions: Add milk (rice, soy, or cow's), cinnamon, and/or walnuts for additional flavor and protein.

Preparation time: 50 to 65 minutes

Servings: four ¾ cup servings

Nutritional analysis (per serving): Calories, 190; fat, 2.5 g; cholesterol, 0 mg; sodium, 40 mg; carbohydrates, 36 g; sugar, 5 g; fiber, 5 g; protein, 6 g; calcium, 15 mg

Additional calories (with maple syrup or honey, per teaspoon): 20

Oat and Amaranth Hot Cereal

This is a hearty breakfast of whole grains. It is high in fiber, amino acids, minerals, and B vitamins. The blueberries add the benefits of phytonutrients (plant nutrients) and antioxidants; walnuts add omega-3 essential fatty acids. This breakfast will energize you for the whole morning. The longer it cooks, the creamier it will be. This recipe can be stored in the refrigerator to be reheated for a quick breakfast.

¼ cup amaranth

½ cup steel-cut oats

3½ cups water

Dash of sea salt

½ cup milk (nonfat milk, soymilk, or rice milk)

½ cup blueberries (frozen or fresh)

3 tablespoons walnuts, in pieces or coarsely chopped

Maple syrup, to taste

Using a fine strainer, rinse amaranth in cool water. Put oats and amaranth into a medium saucepan with water and salt. Bring to a boil; reduce heat to simmer (to a point where the grains are still moving). Add milk. Stir to prevent grains from sticking to the pot. Cover and cook for 25 to 30 minutes. Add blueberries and walnuts 5 minutes before end of cooking time. Serve hot. Add maple syrup to desired sweetness.

As an alternative to using amaranth in the recipe, replace it with an equal amount of steel-cut oats. Cover and cook for 30 to 35 minutes or follow the package instructions for cooking steel-cut oats.

Tip: Store leftovers in a covered container in the refrigerator, and reheat for a quick breakfast. The mixture will have thickened, so stir in additional liquid (water or milk) when reheating to thin to the desired texture. Will keep for up to 4 days.

Preparation time: 35 to 40 minutes

Servings: three ¾ cup servings

Nutritional analysis (per serving using soymilk): Calories, 240; fat, 9 g; cholesterol, 0 mg; sodium, 70 mg; carbohydrates, 33 g; sugar, 4 g; fiber, 7 g; protein, 9 g; calcium, 60 mg

Additional calories (with maple syrup, per teaspoon): 20

Leafy Greens Sauté

Leafy greens are the most overlooked vegetable in the produce section. They are especially high in calcium and rich in antioxidants. This quick, easy recipe will round out any meal.

8 cups chopped raw greens (kale, chard, collards, spinach, or
    a mix of these)
1 to 2 tablespoons extra-virgin olive oil
1 tablespoon minced garlic
½ to 1 teaspoon balsamic vinegar
½ teaspoon soy sauce or salt, to taste

For greens with tough stems, pull the leaves off the stem and discard stems before washing. Wash greens in a basin or sink filled with cold water: submerge the greens, and swish in water. Repeat if water is murky. Drain well in a colander. Chop into approximately 2-inch pieces.

Heat oil on medium-high in a large skillet or wok. Add garlic and sauté for 15 seconds. Add greens and toss frequently in the skillet. When all greens have turned bright green and begun to wilt, remove from heat. Sprinkle with vinegar and soy sauce. Toss gently and serve hot.

Serving suggestion: Serve with baked salmon and brown basmati rice.

Preparation time: 15 minutes

Servings: four ½ cup servings

Nutritional analysis (per serving prepared with kale): Calories, 100; fat, 4.5 g; cholesterol, 0 mg; sodium, 100 mg; carbohydrates, 14 g; sugar, 3 g; fiber, 3 g; protein, 5 g; calcium, 200 mg

Wholesome Blueberry Muffins

These muffins can be eaten for breakfast or an on-the-go snack. They are high in fiber, low-fat, and full of antioxidants provided by the blueberries. In addition, they are dairy- and egg-free. The muffins have just the right level of sweetness.

½ cup sucanat (dehydrated cane juice)

3 tablespoons organic canola oil

¼ cup apple sauce, unsweetened

¾ cup plain soymilk

1 teaspoon apple-cider vinegar

1 teaspoon vanilla extract

1½ cups whole-wheat pastry flour

½ cup wheat germ

3 tablespoons aluminum-free baking powder

½ teaspoon salt

1½ cup blueberries (frozen is OK)

Preheat oven to 350°F. Oil muffin tins or line with paper baking cups.

In a small bowl, mix together the sucanat, canola oil, apple sauce, soymilk, apple-cider vinegar, and vanilla.

In a separate large bowl, combine dry ingredients (flour, wheat germ, baking powder, and salt); mix well. Make a well in the center of the dry ingredients and pour in wet ingredients from the small bowl. Stir to mix thoroughly (do not overmix). Carefully fold blueberries into the batter.

Spoon the batter into the muffin tins; fill to about halfway. Bake muffins on the center rack of the oven for 20 to 25 minutes.

Tip: As an alternative to using sucanat, replace it with the same amount of maple syrup or honey and add an additional 2 to 3 tablespoons of whole-wheat pastry flour to offset the moisture from the liquid sweetener.

Preparation time: 35 to 40 minutes

Servings: 14 to 18 muffins, depending on size

Nutritional analysis (per muffin): Calories, 106; fat, 3.5 g; cholesterol, 0 mg; sodium, 282 mg; carbohydrates, 18 g; sugar, 7 g; fiber, 2 g; protein, 3 g

Garbanzo Bean and Quinoa Salad

Quinoa (pronounced "KEEN-wa") is an ancient grain of the Incas, a native tribe of South America. It is a unique whole grain because it is a complete protein (contains all eight essential amino acids). Quinoa is also rich in calcium and iron. This salad is high in protein from both the quinoa and garbanzo beans, and high in fiber.

Salad:

6 cups water

1¼ cups quinoa

Dash of sea salt

½ cup carrots, chopped

1 cup garbanzo beans, cooked (or canned) and drained

1 cup fresh parsley, chopped

For dressing:

1 clove garlic, minced

4 tablespoons brown-rice vinegar

2 tablespoons extra-virgin olive oil

2 tablespoons soy sauce

Bring water to a boil in a large pot. In the meantime, in a fine-mesh strainer, rinse quinoa with warm water. Carefully add salt and quinoa to boiling water. Boil for 8 to 10 minutes. Remove from heat and drain quinoa through a large strainer similar to the way you would prepare pasta.

In a large bowl, combine dressing ingredients. Add carrots, garbanzo beans, parsley, and quinoa; toss well. Serve alone or on a bed of lettuce greens at room temperature or chilled.

Preparation time: 15 to 20 minutes

Servings: 6

Nutritional analysis (per serving): Calories, 250; fat, 8 g; cholesterol, 0 mg; sodium, 425 mg; carbohydrates, 34 g; sugar, 3 g; fiber, 12 g; protein, 9 g; calcium, 48 mg

Colorful Tossed Salad

This is not your usual green salad. This recipe will inspire you to expand your color palate to create interesting salads. The more colorful, the higher the level of carotenes—the natural antioxidants with cancer-fighting and health-promoting benefits. If you add protein, this salad is a complete meal. Note: A well-tossed salad requires less dressing.

Lettuce (a combination of romaine,
	green leafy, red leafy, and spinach), torn into
	bite-sized pieces
Purple/red cabbage, thinly sliced or shredded
Carrots, thinly sliced or grated
Red, yellow, and/or green bell peppers, sliced
Red onion, thinly sliced
Tomatoes (cherry, grape, red, yellow, or purple)
Fruit choices: Red or green grapes, chopped
	apples, or pears

Protein choices: Grilled chicken breast, fish (canned or cooked); sesame, sunflower, or pumpkin seeds; walnuts, almonds

Wash all fruits and vegetables and shake off excess water. Put all ingredients into a large bowl. Toss well with a dressing of your choice.

Suggested salad dressing combinations: Experiment with various proportions of the following ingredients:

Oils: Olive, flaxseed, walnut

Vinegar: Balsamic, apple cider, red wine, lemon juice, orange juice

Fresh herbs and spices: Basil, oregano, thyme, dill, garlic, pepper, lemon or orange zest, salsa

Tips: Always have a washed and ready-to-eat salad on hand in the refrigerator. Prepare salad with all the vegetables, but keep wet ingredients such as tomatoes or cut fruit separate until ready to eat; they will wilt the salad. Use a salad spinner to dry the vegetables. Store the dried vegetables in an airtight container or ziplock bag in the refrigerator. Store the wet ingredients (cut tomatoes and fruit) separately until ready to eat, and then toss with dry ingredients, protein (if used), and dressing. The salad will keep for up to 5 days depending on the freshness of the ingredients.

Note: Nutritional analysis and servings not provided because of ingredient options presented. To figure out the nutritional analysis of your salad, see the USDA National Nutrient Database online at www.nal.usda.gov/fnic/food comp/search/.

Roasted Vegetables

This is a very flexible recipe; you can pick and choose the vegetables that you want. Be aware that some vegetables take longer to cook than others. Root vegetables such

as carrots and potatoes take the longest to cook. Start with the vegetables that take the longest to cook, and then add the faster-cooking vegetables afterward.

Use a selection of these recommended vegetables:

Potatoes	Sweet peppers (red, yellow, and/
Sweet potatoes or yams	or orange)
Carrots	Eggplant
Parsnips	Mushrooms
Brussels sprouts	Zucchini
	Onions

Use a selection of these recommended seasonings:

Garlic	Herbs: rosemary, basil,
Salt	oregano (be creative;
Pepper	dried herbs usually
Balsamic vinegar	work best)

Required ingredient:
Olive oil (use enough to coat vegetables)

Optional ingredient:
Chicken or vegetable broth

Preheat oven to 425°F. Cut vegetables into 1½- to 2-inch pieces. In a large bowl, toss vegetables to coat in olive oil, herbs, and seasonings. Put in a shallow baking pan. Place in preheated oven, tossing frequently to brown all sides. Bake until vegetables are cooked to desired tenderness. Add a few tablespoons of chicken or vegetable broth if pan becomes too dry. Add salt to taste and serve.

Note: Vegetable placement may need to be staged by putting longer-cooking vegetables in first. If using onions, put them in at the very beginning so they will caramelize.

Preparation time: Approximately 25 to 40 minutes (incl. vegetable cutting)

Note: Nutritional analysis and servings not provided because of ingredient options presented. To figure out the nutritional analysis of your roasted vegetables, see the USDA National Nutrient Database online at www.nal.usda. gov/fnic/foodcomp/search/.

Lemon Ginger Salmon

I came to fully appreciate salmon when I moved to the Pacific Northwest. Salmon is a big a part of the Pacific Northwest diet and can be a healthy part of anyone's diet. Besides being delicious, salmon is nutritionally superior for its high omega-3 essential fatty acid and low saturated fat content. Salmon requires very little seasoning to taste good. This recipe has a bit of an Asian flair with the mild flavors of the ginger and soy.

1-pound salmon fillet (choose wild over farm-raised)

For marinade:
1 teaspoon grated ginger
1 tablespoon soy sauce
3 tablespoons lemon juice
1 scallion, finely sliced
¼ cup water

Prepare salmon: Rinse salmon fillet under cold water. Pat salmon dry with a paper towel. Run fingers along fillet to feel for bones. Using a small pair of clean pliers, pull bones from fillet and discard. Lay salmon skin side down in a baking pan.

Prepare marinade: In a small bowl, peel and discard skin from ginger. Grate the peeled ginger on a ceramic grater (a fine cheese grater will work too). Pour soy sauce and lemon juice over grated ginger to loosen it from the grater into the bowl. Add scallion. Mix well.

Marinate salmon: Pour marinade over salmon; cover and refrigerate for 25 to 30 minutes.

Cook salmon: Preheat oven to 400°F. Pour ¼ cup water around the salmon. Place baking pan with the marinated salmon on the middle rack in oven. Bake for approximately 15 to 20 minutes, checking frequently until salmon begins to flake on the outside. Remove from heat, spoon marinade sauce from pan onto salmon, and serve hot.

Serving suggestion: Serve on a bed of brown basmati rice, with sautéed greens and a small salad.

Preparation time: 40 to 50 minutes (includes marinating time)

Servings: four 4-ounce servings

Nutritional analysis (per serving): Calories, 162; fat, 4.5 g; cholesterol, 60 mg; sodium, 290 mg; carbohydrates, 1 g; sugar, 0 g; fiber, 0 g; protein, 27 g; calcium: 52 mg

Tofu and Mixed Vegetable Stir-fry

This is a quick way to prepare vegetables with an Asian flavor without too much fuss. If you decide to omit the tofu, use this as a side dish to serve with a protein food. If you use tofu, it is a complete meal. The Vegetarian Stir-Fry Sauce can be found in most Asian markets and in the ethnic food section of some grocery stores; otherwise, soy sauce or tamari will do just fine.

1 tablespoon olive or canola oil

12 ounces firm tofu, cut into 1-inch cubes

1 small onion, chopped

1 clove of garlic, minced

1 medium head of broccoli, cut into flowerets

1 cup mixed vegetables (use a combination of chopped red
  bell peppers, mushrooms, snow peas, and/or carrots)

Water or vegetable broth

3 tablespoons Vegetarian Stir-Fry Sauce, or 2 tablespoons soy
  sauce or tamari

1 teaspoon toasted sesame seeds

Heat half of oil on high in a large skillet or wok. Add tofu and decrease heat to medium-high; sauté until tofu is browned. Remove tofu from pan. Heat remaining oil on medium-high, and add onion and garlic; sauté until onion is soft. Add broccoli and other vegetables, and reduce heat to medium. Sauté until vegetables reach desired tenderness. Add water or broth if pan becomes too dry. Add browned tofu and Vegetarian Stir-Fry Sauce. Mix well. Sprinkle with sesame seeds and serve hot.

Preparation time: 20 minutes

Servings: 4

Nutritional analysis (per serving with soy sauce): Calories, 130; fat, 7 g; cholesterol, 0 mg; sodium, 530 mg; carbohydrates, 9 g; sugar, 4 g; fiber, 2 g; protein, 8 g; calcium, 150 g

Appendix C

Healthy Bride Travel Workout

This is a workout for those of you who travel and would like an easy workout to take with you on the road.

This workout includes:

Body Weight Exercises

Standing or Walking Lunges   Abdominal Crunches

Standing Squats   Oblique Curls

Bridges   Reverse Crunches

Tricep Dips   Back Extensions

Modified or Full Body Push-ups

Band Exercises

Standing Rows

Standing Chest Press

Bicep Curls

Before performing the following workout, make sure you warm up for five full minutes by walking, marching, or using a cardio machine. Most hotels and cruise ships have a workout room—a great option for staying on track with your exercise program.

Body Weight Exercises
Standing or Walking Lunges (2 sets of 15 reps per leg)

1. From a standing position, take a giant step forward with one foot and land on your heel.

2. Bend both knees, slowly lowering your hips to the floor. Make sure your front knee is directly over your ankle. You should be able to see your toes at all times.

3. Bend your back knee so that it is near but not touching the floor. Keep your weight distributed over your entire front foot.

4. Push off with your back foot and bring it forward to standing position.

5. Continue walking forward in this fashion, switching legs with each step.

Standing Squats (2 sets of 15 reps)

1. Stand with your legs shoulder width apart. Focus all your body weight on your heels.

2. Stick your buttocks out behind you and lower your body by bending your knees toward the floor. Lower your body until your thighs are parallel to the floor. Make sure you can see your toes past your knees at the lowest point in the exercise.

3. Repeat.

Bridges (2 sets of 15 reps)

1. Lie on your back.

2. Bend your knees. Your feet should be flat on the floor, 12–18 inches away from your buttocks.

3. Keep your arms flat on the floor and at your sides throughout this exercise.

4. Keep your head resting on a mat.

5. Lift your hips until your body core (your trunk region) raises up off the floor. Only your shoulders and head should be touching the floor at this point. (Before starting this exercise, you can place a towel under your shoulder blades for extra cushioning.)

6. After lifting your hips as high as you can go, hold the position for 10 seconds, then slowly lower yourself back to the floor.

7. Repeat.

Tricep Dips (no band needed; 2 sets of 15–20 reps)

1. Sit on the edge of a bench, step, or sturdy chair.

2. Position your hands beside your body on the edge of the bench (or step or chair), your fingers facing forward.

3. Lift your buttocks off the bench and lower your buttocks toward the floor by bending your arms at the

elbows. Make sure you stay perpendicular to the ground, and keep your back straight. Don't push your hips forward.

4. Lift yourself back up by straightening your arms. Keep your arms close to your body throughout the movement.

Modified or Full Body Push-ups (2 sets of 10)

1. Get into bent-knee push-up position with your hands and knees on the floor. Make sure that your hands are under your shoulders, your back is flat, and your hips are parallel to the floor. (For full body push-ups, get into the same position, except keep your toes, rather than your knees, on the floor and keep your entire body in a straight line.)

2. Lower your chin to the floor, going as low as you can.

3. Return to start position.

Abdominal Crunches (20 total)

1. Lie on the floor with your knees bent and feet flat. Your hands should rest on your thighs, or place your fingers at your temples.

2. Squeeze your abdominal muscles, push your back flat, and rise high enough so that your hands touch the tops of your knees (if you started with them on your thighs) or your shoulder blades come off the floor (if

you placed your fingers at your temples). Don't pull with your neck or head. Keep your lower back on the floor.

3. Return to start position.

4. Repeat.

Oblique Curls (20 total)

1. Lie on the floor with your knees bent and feet flat.

2. Place your fingers on your temples or rest them on your shoulders.

3. Squeeze your abdominal muscles, pushing your back flat, as you cross your left shoulder toward your right hip.

4. Return to start position.

5. Repeat, crossing your right shoulder to your left hip.

6. Return to start position.

7. Repeat.

Reverse Crunches (20 total)

1. Lie on your back on the floor.

2. Raise your feet in the air, legs straight, with your soles are facing the ceiling.

3. Extend your arms out to either side.

4. Lift your hips off the ground, straight up, feet move toward your head. This should only be a small movement.

5. Return to start position.

6. Repeat.

Back Extensions (20 total)

1. Lie flat on the floor, face down.

2. Extend your arms straight above your head, keeping them on the floor.

3. Raise your right arm and left leg at the same time, lifting them as high as you feel comfortable.

4. Hold for the count of three, and then lower your arm and leg.

5. Raise your left arm and right leg at the same time, lifting as high as you feel comfortable.

6. Hold to the count of three, and then lower your arm and leg.

7. Repeat.

Band Exercises

You will need a door attachment for the following resistance-band exercises.

Standing Rows (2 sets of 15–20 reps)

1. Attach an exercise band to a chest-high attachment point.

2. Face the attachment point. Stand far enough away that the band is taut.

3. Take a band handle in each hand, keeping your wrists straight and your palms facing each other. Do not shrug your shoulders.

4. At all times, your feet should be shoulder width apart with your knees slightly bent. Bend your knees enough to keep a solid stance. Pull the band toward you, keeping your elbows at your side and moving your hands toward your chest. The movement should be slow and steady.

5. Release back to full extension at the same speed you pulled the bands toward you.

6. Repeat.

Standing Chest Press (2 sets of 15–20 reps)

1. Attach the bands behind you at approximately chest height. (To do this, use a door attachment or put the bands around a stationary object.)

2. With a band handle in each hand, walk away from the attachment point until the band is taut. Keep a staggered stance to give you more stability. Stand up straight, and keep your abdominal muscles tight, with your chest up, palms facing the floor, elbows at a 90-degree angle at chest height.

3. Press the band handles forward in a steady pushing motion, while keeping your wrists straight.

4. Press to the end of your range of motion or until your hands meet in front of you at chest level. You may need to adjust your distance from the attachment point so that your arms can move through the full range of motion.

5. Release the push, and return backward through these steps until you reach your starting point.

6. Repeat.

Bicep Curls (2 sets of 15-20 reps)

1. Stand with your feet shoulder width apart and your knees slightly bent. If you're using a resistance band, stand on the center of the band with one foot.

2. Hold one band handle in each hand. Keep your hands at your sides, with your palms facing up.

3. Curl both arms up toward your shoulders, moving only from your elbow. Make sure you do not move

your shoulder joint. At the "top" of the curl, your palm should be facing your bicep.

4. Lower your arms back to start position.

5. Repeat.

Bibliography

Part One: Starting Out

ACSM Guidelines for Exercise Testing and Prescription, 6th ed. Philadelphia: Lippincott, Williams, & Wilkins, 2000.

American Heart Association. www.americanheart.org

Dunn, A. L., B. H. Marcus, J. B. Kampert, M. E. Garcia, H. W. Kohl, and S. N. Blair. "Reduction in Cardiovascular Disease Risk Factors: 6-month Results from Project Active." *Preventive Medicine,* 26 (1997): 883–92.

Glanz, K., R. E. Patterson, A. R. Kristal, C. C. DeClemente, J. Heimendinger, L. Linnan, et al. "Stages of Change in Adopting Healthy Diets: Fat, Fiber, and Correlates of Nutrient Intake." *Health Education Quarterly*, vol. 21 (1994): 499–519.

Grimley, D. M., G. E. Riley, J. M. Bellis, and J. O. Prochaska. "Assessing the Stages of Change and Decision-making for Contraceptive Use for the Prevention of Pregnancy, Sexually Transmitted Diseases, and Acquired Immunodeficiency Syndrome." *Health Education Quarterly*, vol. 29 (1993): 455–70.

Hellman, E. A. "Use of the Stages of Change in Exercise Adherence Model Among Older Adults with a Cardiac Diagnosis." *Journal of Cardiopulmonary Rehabilitation*, vol. 17 (1997): 145–55.

Manson, J. E., H. Tosteson, P. M. Ridker, et al. "The Primary Prevention of Myocardial Infarction." *New England Journal of Medicine*, vol. 326 (1992): 1406–13.

Marcus, B. H., S. W. Banspach, R. C. Lefebvre, J. S. Rossi, R. A. Carleton, and D. B. Abrams. "Using the Stages of Change Model to Increase the Adoption of Physical Activity Among Community Participants." *American Journal of Health Promotion*, vol. 6 (1992): 424–29.

Marcus, B. H., W. Rakowski, and R. S. Rossi. "Assessing Motivational Readiness and Decision-making for Exercise." *Health Psychology*, 11 (1992): 257–61.

Nash, Joyce D., Ph.D. *The New Maximize Your Body Potential: Lifetime Skills for Successful Weight Managewment.* Palo Alto, CA: Bull Publishing, 1997.

Physical Fitness Specialist Manual, rev. ed. Dallas: The Cooper Institute, 2005.

"The President's Council on Physical Fitness and Sports." Department of Health and Human Services. www.fitness.gov.

Prochaska, J. O., W. F. Velicer, J. S. Rossi, M. G. Goldstein, B. H. Marcus, W. Rakowski, et al. "Stages of Change and Decisional Balance for 12 Problem Behaviors." *Health Psychology*, vol. 13 (1994): 39–46.

Prochaska, J. O., and C. C. DiClemente. "The Stages and Processes of Self-change in Smoking: Towards an Integrative Model of Change." *Journal of Consulting and Clinical Psychology*, vol. 51, 390–95.

Part Two: Healthy Bride Fitness Program

ACSM Guidelines for Exercise Testing and Prescription, 6th ed. Philadelphia: Lippincott, Williams, & Wilkins, 2000.

ACSM's Resource Manual for Guidelines for Exercise Testing and Prescription, 4th ed. Philadelphia: Lippincott, Williams, & Wilkins, 2001.

Borg, G. V. "Psychological Basis of Perceived Exertion." *Medicine & Science in Sports & Exercise*, vol. 14 (1982): 377–81.

Chek, Paul. *How to Eat, Move and Be Healthy.* San Diego: C.H.E.K. Institute, 2004.

Goldenberg, Lorne, and Peter Twist. *Strength Ball Training.* Champaign, IL: Human Kinetics, 2002.

Journal of the American College of Cardiology, vol. 37, no. 1 (2001): pp. 153–56.

Golding, Lawrence A., et al. *The Y's Way to Physical Fitness*, 3rd ed. (Champaign, IL: Human Kinetics, 1989), 106–08, 119–24.

Morris, Mike, and Stephanie Morris. *CORE Instructor Certification Manual*. Venice, CA: Resist-A-Ball, Inc., 2001.

Nieman, David C. *Exercise Testing and Prescription*, 4th ed. Mountain View, CA: Mayfield Publishing, 1999.

"The President's Council on Physical Fitness and Sports." Department of Health and Human Services. www.fitness.gov.

Tanaka, H., K. D. Monahan, and D. R. Seals. "Age-predicted Maximal Heart Rate Revisited." *Journal of the American College of Cardiology*, vol. 37 (2001): 153–58.

Part Three: Healthy Bride Nutrition Program

ACE Personal Trainer Manual, 3rd ed. (San Diego: American Council on Exercise, 2003), 127, 129, 141.

American Dietetic Association. "Dietary Reference Intakes Released for Carbohydrates, Fats, Protein, Fiber, and Physical Activity." *Dietetics in Practice*, vol. 2, no. 2 (2002).

American Dietetic Association. "Food and Nutrition Information." www.eatright.org/Public/NutritionInformation/92.cfm.

Cattlemen's Beef Board and National Cattlemen's Beef Association. "Nutrient Comparisons of Meat, Poultry, and Seafood." www.beef-nutrition.com/Udocs/Nutrient%20Comps%20for%20bn_18-215.pdf.

Caughlin, Goldie. *Still Eating Square Meals?* Seattle: Foodworks! Nutrition Education Program of Puget Consumers Co-op, n.d.

Center for Food Safety and Applied Nutrition. "Questions and Answers about Trans Fat Nutrition Labeling." U.S. Food and Drug Administration. www.cfsan.fda.gov/~dms/qatrans2.html.

Center for Science in the Public Interest. "CSPI's Guide to Food Additives." www.cspinet.org/reports/chemcuisine.htm.

Department of Health and Human Services and U.S. Department of Agriculture. "Dietary Guidelines for 2005." www.healthierus.gov/dietaryguidelines/.

"Government Releases Dietary Guidelines Committee Report." *ADA Times* (Sept./Oct. 2004): 1, 9-10.

Holt, S. H., N. Sandona, and J. C. Brand-Miller. "The Effects of Sugar-free vs. Sugar-rich Beverages on Feelings of Fullness and Subsequent Food Intake." *International Journal of Food Sciences and Nutrition* (January 2000): 59-71.

Khan, Sumiya, M.S., R.D. *Your Guide to Eating Out the Healthy Way*. Kent, WA: Community Health Centers of King County, 2004.

Lavin, J. H., S. J. French, and N. W. Read. "The Effect of Sucrose- and Aspartame-sweetened Drinks on Energy Intake, Hunger, and Food Choice of Female, Moderately Restrained Eaters." *International Journal of Obesity and Related Metabolic Disorders* (January 1997): 37-42.

Mahan, L. Kathleen, M.S., R.D., C.D.E., and Sylvia Escott-Stump, M.A., R.D., L.D.N. *Krause's Food, Nutrition, and Diet Therapy*, 10th ed. (New York: WB Saunders Company, 2000): 33-63.

Murray, Michael T., N.D. *Encyclopedia of Nutritional Supplements*. (New York: Prima Publishing, 1996): 119-26, 239-78.

Roberts, Arthur J., M.D., Mary E. O'Brien, M.D., and Genell Subak-Sharpe. *Nutraceuticals: The Complete Encyclopedia of Supplements, Herbs, Vitamins, and Healing Foods.* (New York: The Berkley Publishing Group, 2001): 219-21, 237-38, 241-42.

Robinson, Dorene D., R.D., C.N., ed. *Beyond Fitness: Nutrition and Healthy Strategies for a Better Life*. Bellevue, WA: Peak Performance, 1999.

U.S. Department of Agriculture. "Nutrient Database for Standard Reference." www.nal.usda.gov/fnic/foodcomp/search/.

U.S. Environmental Protection Agency. "Consumption Advice: Fish Advisories." www.epa.gov/waterscience/fish/advisory.html.

Willett, Walter, M.D. *Eat, Drink, and Be Healthy: The Harvard Medical School Guide to Healthy Eating*. New York: Free Press, 2003.

Part Four: Stress and the Healthy Bride

Danksin, David G. "Meditation and Relaxation." Texas Woman's University Self-help Library. www.twu.edu/o-sl/counseling/Self-Help039.html.

University of Florida Counseling Center. "Relaxation Exercise." www.counsel.ufl.edu/selfHelp/relaxation.asp.

Part Five: Beyond Bridal

Nash, Joyce D., Ph.D. *The New Maximize Your Body Potential: Lifetime Skills for Successful Weight Management*. Palo Alto, CA: Bull Publishing, 1997.

About the Authors

CHRISTI MASI founded The Healthy Bride and Seattle Wedding Trainer to focus on training women for one of life's greatest pivotal moments. Although her focus is training brides for their wedding day, she loves to work with any woman who wants to further her health and fitness. Christi holds both ACSM-HFI and NSCA-CPT certifications and has a BA in Psychology from the University of Washington. Since 1994 Christi has been successfully training women for life firsts: triathlons, 10K races, summits of Mt. Rainier, weddings, class reunions, and numerous weight-loss goals. Christi enjoys working with committed individuals to make their dreams come true.

SHERI K. MAR, M.S., C.N., is a professional nutritionist with an advanced degree in nutrition from Bastyr University. She abandoned the high-tech world of Silicon Valley to pursue a career in nutrition in Seattle. She is also an ACE-certified personal trainer and a Lifetime Fitness Program-certified instructor, promoting physical activity among older adults. Sheri has won awards for her volunteer work providing nutrition education to senior and disabled citizens. An enthusiastic modern dancer, Sheri loves cooking and keeping fit, and encouraging good health and proper nutrition in others.

From this day forward, In fitness and in health. . .

On your wedding day, you want to look and feel your best. You've seen those other bridal workouts with extreme exercise programs and crash diets. *The Healthy Bride Guide* combats flash-in-the-pan programs with a fitness and nutrition program geared not just to trimming your waistline for your Big Day, but also to jump-starting a healthy lifestyle for you and your new husband.

The HEALTHY BRIDE program includes:

➔ Personal health assessment to track your starting point and your progress

➔ Exercise program to improve strength, cardiovascular fitness, and flexibility

➔ In-depth guide to proper nutrition and weight loss (Guess what? You *should* eat carbs *and* fat!)

➔ Stress management exercises and advice to get you through pre-wedding mania

➔ Travel workout program (for exercising in confined spaces)

➔ Tips on how to fight the backslide

➔ And much more . . .

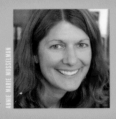

Christi Masi is a Seattle-based personal trainer who works with women to prepare for pivotal life moments, most notably with brides-to-be before their weddings. She is the founder of The (Seattle) Wedding Trainer and The Healthy Bride™—both devoted to working with women committed to improving their health and fitness.

Sheri Mar is a certified nutritionist with a master in nutrition degree from Bastyr University. She lives in Seattle.

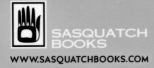

SASQUATCH BOOKS

WWW.SASQUATCHBOOKS.COM

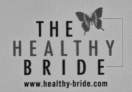

THE HEALTHY BRIDE

www.healthy-bride.com

1-57061-461-X $19.95 U.S.

51995

9 781570 614613

From this day forward, In fitness and in health. . .

On your wedding day, you want to look and feel your best. You've seen those other bridal workouts with extreme exercise programs and crash diets. *The Healthy Bride Guide* combats flash-in-the-pan programs with a fitness and nutrition program geared not just to trimming your waistline for your Big Day, but also to jump-starting a healthy lifestyle for you and your new husband.

The HEALTHY BRIDE program includes:

→ Personal health assessment to track your starting point and your progress

→ Exercise program to improve strength, cardiovascular fitness, and flexibility

→ In-depth guide to proper nutrition and weight loss (Guess what? You *should* eat carbs *and* fat!)

→ Stress management exercises and advice to get you through pre-wedding mania

→ Travel workout program (for exercising in confined spaces)

→ Tips on how to fight the backslide

→ And much more . . .

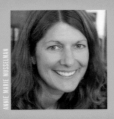

ANNIE MARIE MUSSELMAN

Christi Masi is a Seattle-based personal trainer who works with women to prepare for pivotal life moments, most notably with brides-to-be before their weddings. She is the founder of The (Seattle) Wedding Trainer and The Healthy Bride™—both devoted to working with women committed to improving their health and fitness.

Sheri Mar is a certified nutritionist with a master in nutrition degree from Bastyr University. She lives in Seattle.

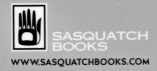

SASQUATCH BOOKS

WWW.SASQUATCHBOOKS.COM

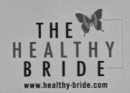

THE HEALTHY BRIDE

www.healthy-bride.com

1-57061-461-X $19.95 U.S.

51995

9 781570 614613